Dr. Ann's Weigh Less for Life

21 KEY STRATEGIES TO LASTING WEIGHT LOSS

By Ann G. Kulze, MD

Editorial Staff

Author: Ann G. Kulze, MD

Executive Editor: David Hunnicutt, PhD

Managing Editor: Brittanie Leffelman, MS

Contributing Editor: Elizabeth Kulze, Carie Maguire

Multimedia Designer: Adam Paige

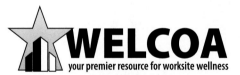

WELCOA
your premier resource for worksite wellness

17002 Marcy Street, Suite 140 | Omaha, NE 68118
PH: 402-827-3590 | FX: 402-827-3594 | welcoa.org

Ann Kulze, MD
CEO
1 Pitt Street
Charleston, SC 29401
PH: 843.329.1238
www.DrAnnwellness.com

All material in this book is provided for educational purposes only. Consult your
personal health care provider regarding any specific opinions or recommendations
related to your symptoms or medical condition.

Table of Contents

About **WELCOA**

The Wellness Council of America (WELCOA) was established as a national not-for-profit organization in the mid 1980s through the efforts of a number of forward-thinking business and health leaders. Drawing on the vision originally set forth by William Kizer, Sr., Chairman Emeritus of Central States Indemnity, and WELCOA founding Directors that included Dr. Louis Sullivan, former Secretary of Health and Human Services, and Warren Buffet, Chairman of Berkshire Hathaway, WELCOA has helped influence the face of workplace wellness in the US.

Today, WELCOA has become one of the most respected resources for workplace wellness in America. With a membership in excess of 5,000 organizations, WELCOA is dedicated to improving the health and well-being of all working Americans. Located in America's heartland, WELCOA makes its national headquarters in one of America's healthiest business communities—Omaha, Nebraska.

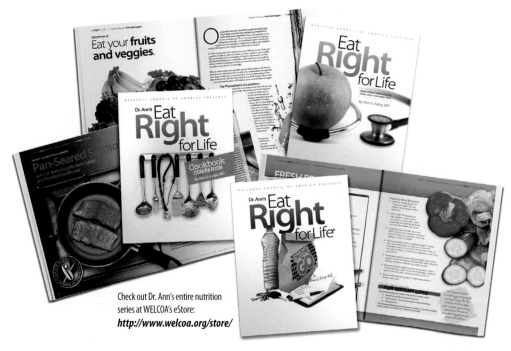

Check out Dr. Ann's entire nutrition series at WELCOA's eStore:
http://www.welcoa.org/store/

About **Ann G. Kulze, MD**

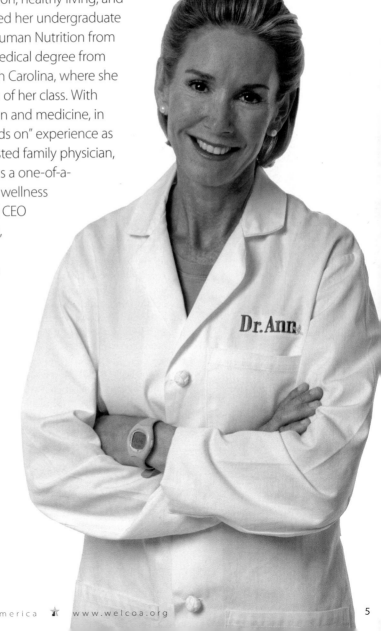

Ann G. Kulze, MD is a renowned authority and motivational speaker on nutrition, healthy living, and disease prevention. She received her undergraduate degree in Food Science and Human Nutrition from Clemson University and her medical degree from the Medical University of South Carolina, where she graduated as the Valedictorian of her class. With formal training in both nutrition and medicine, in addition to her extensive "hands on" experience as a wife, mother of four, and trusted family physician, she has distinguished herself as a one-of-a-kind "real world" nutrition and wellness expert. She is the founder and CEO of the wellness education firm, Just Wellness LLC, and author of several books including the award winning, best-selling *Eat Right for Life®* series.

When she's not writing, researching, or motivating others through her speaking engagements, Dr. Ann lives her wellness message in her native Charleston, SC where she enjoys swimming, running, kayaking, cooking, gardening and spending time with her wonderful family. Learn more at **www.DrAnnWellness.com**.

[FOREWORD]
From Dr. Hunnicutt

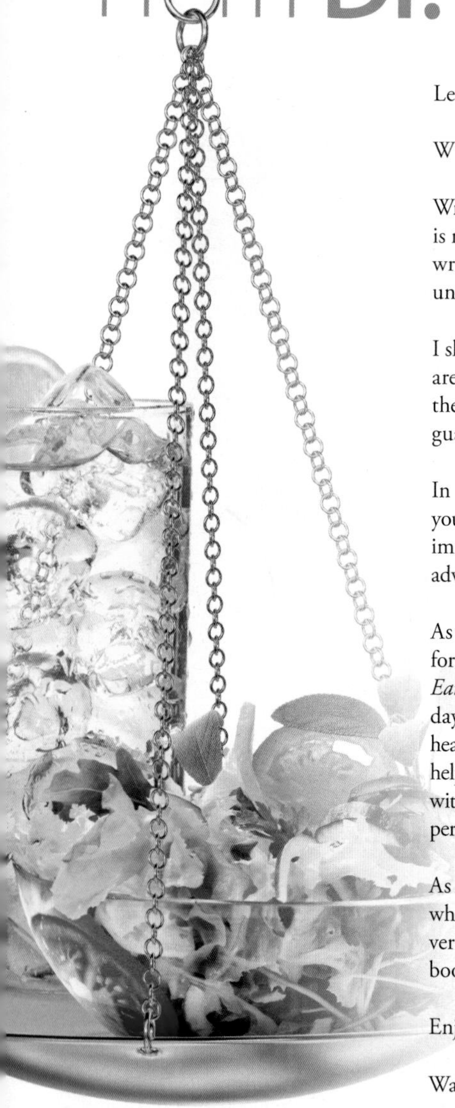

Let's cut to the chase.

When you read this book, you are in for a real treat.

Written by one of the country's foremost experts on nutrition, Dr. Ann Kulze is not only a brilliant physician and health practitioner—she is a great writer. In fact, all of the information that you'll read in this book is easy-to-understand, motivating and fiercely practical.

I share this with you because I am sensitive to the fact that many Americans are suffering from carrying too much weight—and much of the information they desperately need is either inaccurate or impossible to decipher. I can guarantee you that Dr. Ann's approach is neither.

In *Weigh Less for Life,* you will discover 21 key evidence-based strategies to help you experience lasting weight loss. Again each of the strategies is simple and imminently doable. The very best part of it all is this: if you follow Dr. Ann's advice and instruction, you <u>will</u> lose weight—and you <u>will</u> keep it off.

As you move forward on your journey to better health, it's important for you to know that there are three companion books also available. *Eat Right For Life®* lays the foundation for eating well every meal every day. The *Eat Right For Life®: Cookbook Companion* is your key to preparing healthy meals—and enjoying the process. Finally, *Eat Right for Life®: On The Go* helps you to develop a strategy for eating healthfully while eating out. Along with *Weigh Less for Life,* Dr. Ann's compendium of books can help you be the person you want to be.

As you begin the all-important process of changing your personnel behavior when it comes to nutrition, I am confident that you have in your hands a very important part of the solution. Armed with the information in this book, I am confident you can indeed weigh less for life.

Enjoy your journey!

Warmest Regards,

David Hunnicutt, PhD
President
Wellness Council of America

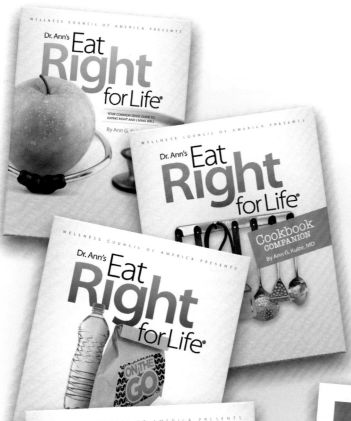

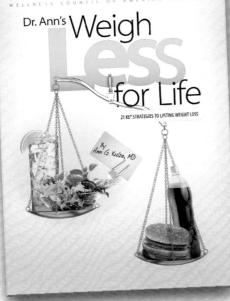

About
DR. DAVID HUNNICUTT

Since his arrival at WELCOA in 1995, David Hunnicutt, PhD has developed countless publications that have been widely adopted in businesses and organizations throughout North America. Known for his ability to make complex issues easier to understand, David has a proven track-record of publishing health and wellness material that helps employees lead healthier lifestyles. David travels extensively advocating better health practices and radically different thinking in organizations of all kinds.

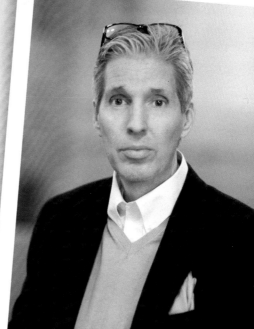

[INTRODUCTION]
Weigh **Less** For Life

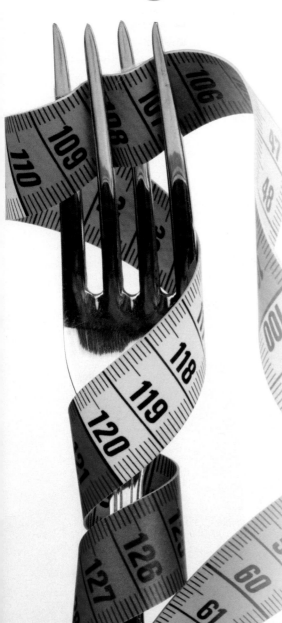

If YOU WANT TO LEARN HOW TO LOSE WEIGHT FOR GOOD AND FEEL GREAT FOR LIFE, THIS BOOK IS FOR YOU. As a physician who has devoted her professional life to empowering people with the knowledge to live the healthiest and longest life, nothing ignites my passion more than teaching people how to lose weight healthfully and permanently. The source of my devotion and enthusiasm for this topic is fundamental. I know that weight control equals disease control and ultimately, quality of life. Other than smoking cessation, keeping your weight in the healthy range or losing weight if you are overweight, provides more built-in disease protection than any other factor under your personal control. In other words, aside from not smoking, weight control is the most powerful personal tool you have to increase your chances of a long, active, and productive life.

This fact of health brings me right to the heart and theme of this entire book—helping you eat less. And helping you succeed in eating less without deprivation, without hunger, and without giving up eating as one of life's greatest pleasures. As someone who is equally passionate about eating for optimal health and eating for pleasure, I promise that the strategies in this book will allow you to enjoy your food and feel deliciously satisfied even as you lose weight and improve your well-being.

Over the past decade I have developed a fascination (I would even call it an obsession), with the science of appetite control and the factors that compel us to seek food and eat. I am convinced, and there is plenty of supportive science, that the primary driver of our bulging bellies and our epidemic levels of obesity is that we eat too much. In other words, the colossal public health crisis we are facing is because so many people have consumed so many excess calories. Although physical activity is invaluable for disease protection and weight maintenance, physical activity levels are not a very reliable predictor of weight gain. It is the calories we take in and the foods we eat that most closely correlate with the weight on the scale. To put it simply, if you are overweight, chances are you got there largely because you consumed too much of the wrong foods.

Thankfully, the body of new science related to hunger, appetite, and what ultimately drives us to eat has exploded over the past two decades. I wrote this book to help you tap into and fully exploit this enormously useful new science so you can weigh less for life. Specifically, I have distilled down the very best of this exciting new science into 21 simple, straightforward, delicious, great-for-you practices that I know you can sink your teeth into permanently. In the pages that follow, I will personally take you through each of these 21 easy and achievable strategies. With each, I will tell you why and how it helps you eat less, and then provide a detailed action plan so you will know exactly how to build it into your life for maximum benefit. In the end, these 21 dietary and behavioral tweaks comprise what the very best science tells us are the very best ways to put YOU in control of your appetite, making YOU the master of how much food you eat. Think of this book as the modern day manifesto for combating hunger and overeating.

Each of the 21 tactics operates through one of three proven paths to help you eat less:

1. Eating the foods that improve appetite control and promote satiety, while avoiding those that drive appetite and perpetuate hunger.

2. Re-engineering or altering your immediate food environments.

3. Adhering to simple mealtime-related behavioral practices.

In stark contrast to most weight loss books, the plan I propose is not a "diet" in any way, shape, or form. Rather it is a comprehensive menu of basic eating tips and lifestyle strategies that leverage the most powerful and effective ways to help you rein in your appetite and empower you to eat less. Each one is intended to be incorporated FOREVER in your life, but at whatever pace works best for you. Meaning you have total control over this completely flexible and 100% adaptable plan. Although I want you to do as you please with the guidance in this book, I do suggest that you begin by selecting just two to four of the eat less commands and adhere to them in a consistent manner until they

become a habit. It is best to begin with those that seem the most doable and relevant to your personal circumstances. Once you have mastered these initial changes and they have become an automatic part of your eating or living, move on to a few more of the eat less strategies. Ideally, continue this practice until you feel confident that you have taken optimal advantage of all of them for your weight control, health, and vitality. I specifically recommend this two-or-three-at-a-time approach because the science supports that most everyone can make a few small, easy changes on a consistent basis. Adhering to a change in your behavior on a regular basis is how new habits are born. This should be your ultimate goal, and how you will find meaningful and lasting success with the information I have provided in this book.

For additional inspiration, I want you to know that as you lose weight by following these eat less directives, you will also be dramatically improving your health. Most of these strategies have dazzling health benefits that extend well beyond your waistline and the scale. In fact, this book could be titled Stay Well for Life because most of the strategies we will cover are also the healthy habits that will invigorate your body, lift your spirits, and radically reduce your chances of becoming ill.

I want you to achieve a healthy body weight, but just as important, I want you to experience the amazing feeling of being able to transform your own health destiny. The path to lasting weight control I have laid out in this book is the way to get there. Better yet, I promise it will be far easier and more enjoyable than most imagine. And best of all—your success will come with a spectacular array of health gifts that will give years to your life and life to your years. So let's get on it!

—*Ann G. Kulze, MD*

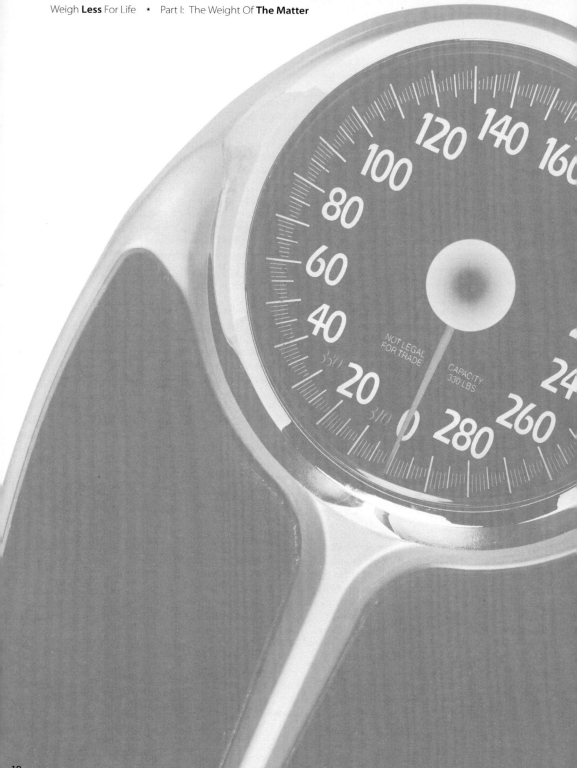

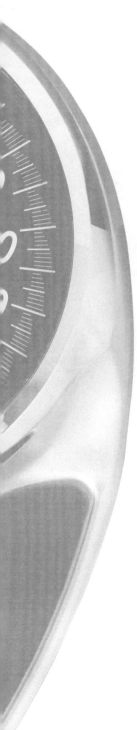

The Weight Of
The Matter

The Weight Of
The Matter

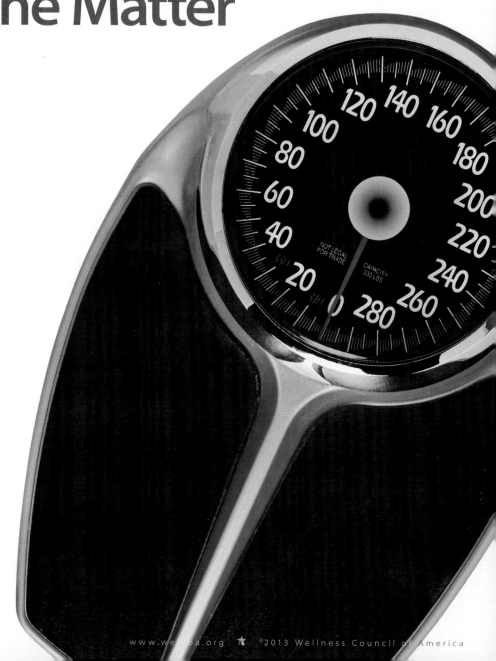

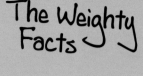

The Weighty Facts

Y OUR BODY WEIGHT IS OF MONUMENTAL IMPORTANCE TO YOUR OVERALL HEALTH AND FUNCTIONALITY. In fact, aside from smoking status, your body weight is the single most powerful predictor of your health. In other words, if you are a non-smoker, the amount of excess fat you carry on your body is the closest thing we have to a crystal ball in determining your future health. This statement is so crucial for your life and well-being that right now—before you read any further—I want you to take a long, mindful pause to let this vital fact sink deep into your psyche.

Thankfully, understanding body fat's all-powerful hold on your health is very straight forward—the more excess fat you have in or on your body, the greater your risks of life-zapping chronic diseases, including three of our biggest killers—cardiovascular disease, cancer, and type 2 diabetes. To see for yourself, please take a look at the 25 adverse health consequences of excess weight gain and obesity noted on the following page. In addition to this list of potentially debilitating health conditions, too much body fat, especially when it reaches obese levels, also has enormous psychosocial consequences including: low self-esteem, depression, social stigmatization, discrimination, and negative body image. Lastly, carrying around a large surplus of body fat can dramatically hinder your functional status, boosting the risk of unemployment, limited physical mobility, disability, absenteeism from work, poor physical fitness, and reduced overall productivity.

In closing, your body weight has a massive impact on your overall health and vitality. The evidence is simply incontrovertible that having too much body fat can turn you into a medical prisoner, rob you of your quality of life, and end your life prematurely.

Despite what you may have heard or read in the popular media, the weight of the evidence is CONVINCING that being overweight (BMI > 25) increases the risk of premature disease AND death. In the most powerful and scientifically rigorous investigation to date, scientists from the National Cancer Institute combined the original data from 19 different studies that tracked body weight and death risk. This evaluation included 1.46 million people followed over about ten years. The results were very clear and very consistent for all age groups—people who were overweight had a greater risk of dying than people who had a normal weight. For every five unit increase in BMI, the risk of death increased by 31%.

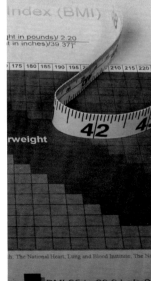

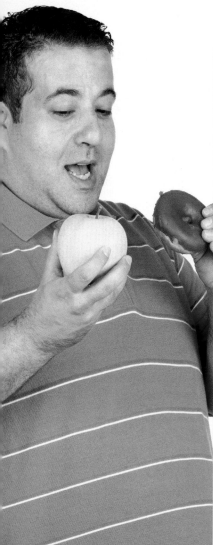

The Health Consequences Of...

EXCESS WEIGHT GAIN AND OBESITY

➤ Heart attacks

➤ Strokes

➤ Heart failure

➤ Abnormal blood fat levels (high cholesterol, high triglycerides, low good cholesterol)

➤ High blood pressure

➤ Prediabetes and type 2 diabetes

➤ Metabolic syndrome

➤ Liver disease (hepatic steatosis)

➤ Adult onset asthma

➤ Gallstones

➤ Sleep apnea

➤ Chronic kidney disease

➤ Osteoarthritis

➤ High uricemia and gout

➤ Infertility

➤ Sexual dysfunction

➤ Cancers of the colon, rectum, breast (post-menopause), esophagus, kidney, uterus, pancreas, and gallbladder

➤ Gastro-esophageal reflux

➤ Pregnancy complications

➤ Fatigue

➤ Poor fitness

➤ Pain

➤ Low vitamin D levels

➤ Depression

➤ Reduced blood flow to the brain

Body Weight And Your Sex Life

According to researchers from Duke University, obesity may dramatically impair sexual quality of life for men and women. In a study involving about 1,200 study subjects who were surveyed about all aspects of their sexual function, 66% of obese study subjects reported sexual difficulties in at least one of four areas vs. just five percent for the normal weight subjects. 42% of obese subjects reported they "sometimes, usually, or always" had sexual dysfunction vs. 1.8% in the normal weight group.

Where Do I Stand?

When trying to gauge where you personally stand in terms of body fat and health risk, there are three relevant metrics for you to know—body mass index (BMI for short), waist size, and how your current weight compares to your weight in your early twenties. In the sections that follow, I will cover how you can determine these three important measurements for yourself and why they matter.

What Is My BMI?

You have likely heard of the term BMI before. Historically, this has been the most commonly used measure in healthcare and medicine to establish how an individual's weight status affects their health risk. BMI is simply a measure of your weight relative to your height. It is calculated by dividing your weight in kilograms by your height in meters squared or:

$$BMI = weight\ (kg)\ /\ height\ (m^2)$$

Thankfully, there are BMI charts available (see chart below) that can do the math for you. First, simply find your height in inches in the left vertical column of the chart. Next, move along the row towards the right until you find your weight in pounds. Finally, refer to the BMI number along the top horizontal column that coincides with your current height and weight. For example, if you are 5 feet 10 inches tall (70 inches in the vertical column) and weigh between 202-206 pounds, your BMI (top horizontal column) is 29.

Current medical definitions of normal weight, overweight, and obese are based on BMI and are as follows:

< 18.5 Underweight | 18.5 – 24.9 Normal | 25.0 – 29.9 Overweight | > 30 Obese

Body Weight Factoids

Relative to normal weight individuals, healthcare costs for obese individuals are $1,429 higher annually.

According to the American Cancer Society, 90,000 cancer deaths could be prevented each year in the U.S. if men and women could keep their weight in the healthy range.

Cancer is the second leading cause of death in the U.S., and according to the American Institute for Cancer Research, obesity causes more than 100,000 new cases of cancer each year in the U.S.

Body Mass Index Table

	Normal						Overweight					Obese										Extreme Obesity														
BMI	19	20	21	22	23	24	25	26	27	28	29	30	31	32	33	34	35	36	37	38	39	40	41	42	43	44	45	46	47	48	49	50	51	52	53	54
Height (inches)															Body Weight (pounds)																					
58	91	96	100	105	110	115	119	124	129	134	138	143	148	153	158	162	167	172	177	181	186	191	196	201	205	210	215	220	224	229	234	239	244	248	253	258
59	94	99	104	109	114	119	124	128	133	138	143	148	153	158	163	168	173	178	183	188	193	198	203	208	212	217	222	227	232	237	242	247	252	257	262	267
60	97	102	107	112	118	123	128	133	138	143	148	153	158	163	168	174	179	184	189	194	199	204	209	215	220	225	230	235	240	245	250	255	261	266	271	276
61	100	106	111	116	122	127	132	137	143	148	153	158	164	169	174	180	185	190	195	201	206	211	217	222	227	232	238	243	248	254	259	264	269	275	280	285
62	104	109	115	120	126	131	136	142	147	153	158	164	169	175	180	186	191	196	202	207	213	218	224	229	235	240	246	251	256	262	267	273	278	284	289	295
63	107	113	118	124	130	135	141	146	152	158	163	169	175	180	186	191	197	203	208	214	220	225	231	237	242	248	254	259	265	270	278	282	287	293	299	304
64	110	116	122	128	134	140	145	151	157	163	169	174	180	186	192	197	204	209	215	221	227	232	238	244	250	256	262	267	273	279	285	291	296	302	308	314
65	114	120	126	132	138	144	150	156	162	168	174	180	186	192	198	204	210	216	222	228	234	240	246	252	258	264	270	276	282	288	294	300	306	312	318	324
66	118	124	130	136	142	148	155	161	167	173	179	186	192	198	204	210	216	223	229	235	241	247	253	260	266	272	278	284	291	297	303	309	315	322	328	334
67	121	127	134	140	146	153	159	166	172	178	185	191	198	204	211	217	223	230	236	242	249	255	261	268	274	280	287	293	299	306	312	319	325	331	338	344
68	125	131	138	144	151	158	164	171	177	184	190	197	203	210	216	223	230	236	243	249	256	262	269	276	282	289	295	302	308	315	322	328	335	341	348	354
69	128	135	142	149	155	162	169	176	182	189	196	203	209	216	223	230	236	243	250	257	263	270	277	284	291	297	304	311	318	324	331	338	345	351	358	365
70	132	139	146	153	160	167	174	181	188	195	202	209	216	222	229	236	243	250	257	264	271	278	285	292	299	306	313	320	327	334	341	348	355	362	369	376
71	136	143	150	157	165	172	179	186	193	200	208	215	222	229	236	243	250	257	265	272	279	286	293	301	308	315	322	329	338	343	351	358	365	372	379	386
72	140	147	154	162	169	177	184	191	199	206	213	221	228	235	242	250	258	265	272	279	287	294	302	309	316	324	331	338	346	353	361	368	375	383	390	397
73	144	151	159	166	174	182	189	197	204	212	219	227	235	242	250	257	265	272	280	288	295	302	310	318	325	333	340	348	355	363	371	378	386	393	401	408
74	148	155	163	171	179	186	194	202	210	218	225	233	241	249	256	264	272	280	287	295	303	311	319	326	334	342	350	358	365	373	381	389	396	404	412	420
75	152	160	168	176	184	192	200	208	216	224	232	240	248	256	264	272	279	287	295	303	311	319	327	335	343	351	359	367	375	383	391	399	407	415	423	431
76	156	164	172	180	189	197	205	213	221	230	238	246	254	263	271	279	287	295	304	312	320	328	336	344	353	361	369	377	385	394	402	410	418	426	435	443

Source: Adapted from *Clinical Guidelines on the Identification, Evaluation, and Treatment of Overweight and Obesity in Adults: The Evidence Report.*

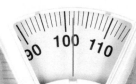

If you are overweight you have a higher risk of premature chronic disease, and the more weight you carry in your mid-section the higher your risk!

Although BMI correlates closely with the risk of weight-related chronic diseases, it does have limitations that are essential to note. First, BMI does not discriminate between lean body tissues (muscle, bone) vs. fat (adipose) tissue. In some cases, individuals that are big boned and very muscular (typically competitive athletes) can have BMI levels in the overweight or even obese range although they have very little body fat. Conversely, some "skinny" individuals can have BMI's in the normal range and still have excess body fat that puts them at significant disease risk. Typically these folks include unfit adults, especially older adults. In fact, the older you are, the less reliable BMI is for assessing health risks.

The second, and arguably the biggest drawback of using BMI to assess health risk, is that it provides no information about the location of excess body fat. As you will learn in the next section, there is now convincing evidence that where you deposit excess fat has major implications for your health.

How Big Is My Belly?
When it comes to body fat and health "where you weigh" is as important, if not more so, than what you weigh. Over the past decade we have learned that the fat that gets deposited within the abdominal cavity (known as visceral fat) behaves in a completely different manner than the subcutaneous fat that gets deposited under the skin in our arms, legs, and buttocks. Unlike subcutaneous fat that functions more so as a simple storage depot for excess calories, visceral fat is a highly active endocrine organ that relentlessly spews out all sorts of nasty, metabolically disruptive chemicals called adipokines. As noted in the graphic on the following page, adipokines have profound and far-reaching harmful effects throughout the body. They include: driving up inflammation, increasing blood pressure, triglycerides, and cholesterol, and promoting insulin resistance and blood clotting. The ultimate fallout from this list of adverse belly fat features are: heart attacks, strokes, high blood pressure, metabolic syndrome, further weight gain, and type 2 diabetes. These are indeed the most common and most closely linked diseases to bulging bellies. The powerful pro-inflammatory adipokines actively secreted by belly fat cells appear to be the red-hot smoking gun that underlies the inextricable bond between large waists and poorer health. And belly fat woes do not end with heart disease and type 2 diabetes. Having a large mid-section has also been linked to colorectal cancer, sleep apnea, cognitive decline, and premature death from all causes.

I want to be sure you note and understand that unlike the more benign subcutaneous fat, even small amounts of belly fat can create metabolic havoc and harm your body. In fact, it appears that "skinny" folks (those with normal BMI's) that have bulging bellies are at a greater risk of heart attack deaths than folks who have a BMI in the obese range! Unfortunately, these skinny, yet centrally obese individuals are quite common. One recent evaluation found that 61% of U.S. adults fell into this category. Meaning, 61% of the study subjects had a normal weight by BMI, but excessive amounts of intra-abdominal fat that put them at risk. As would be expected, the majority of this skinny, yet bigger-bellied bunch also had measurable metabolic abnormalities like high triglycerides and high cholesterol.

Belly Fat **Defined…**

Adipokines: Adverse Cardiometabolic Effects

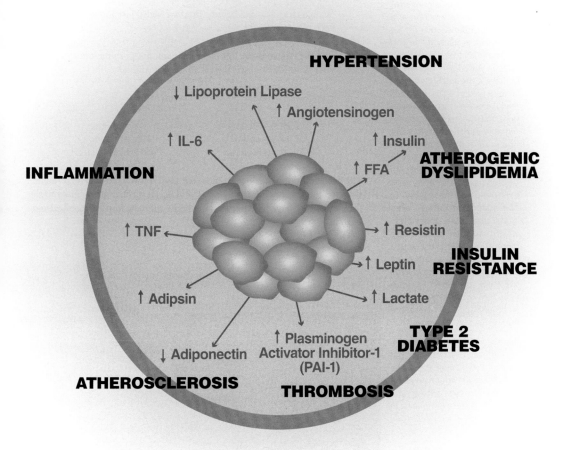

Source: Lyon CJ et al. Endocrinology 2003;144:2195-200. Trayhurn P et al. Br J Nutr. 2004;92:347-55. Eckel RH et al. Lancet. 2005;365:1415-28.

Important News...
ABOUT BELLY FAT

When it comes to body fat and health—it's all about location, location, location. Over the past decade, studies have been piling up showing that the fat deposited within the belly is particularly perilous, especially in terms of metabolic dysfunction and boosting cardiovascular risk. In a landmark evaluation marking the first study to examine death rates in Americans relative to both waist size and body weight (as measured by BMI)—scientists made some eye-opening conclusions. The study included a representative sample of 12,785 adult Americans followed over a 14-year period. Study subjects with a normal weight by BMI, but with large waists as measured by waist to hip ratio, had the highest risk of death from all causes—even higher than those whose body weight put them in the obese range. Relative to those with a normal BMI and a normal waist size, the normal weight, but large waist subjects were 2.75 times more likely to die of cardiovascular disease and 2.08 times more likely to die of all causes.

In a second evaluation that involved over 15,000 cardiac patients followed over about five years, those with a normal weight (by BMI), but excess belly fat were 27% more likely to die relative to obese (by BMI) patients who had less belly fat.

These two reports illustrate the shortcomings of BMI for assessing health risk, especially cardiovascular risk, and hammer home the point that aiming for a smaller waist should take priority over lowering the number on the scale. But for optimal health, it is best to strive for both a normal waist size and a normal body weight by BMI.

For optimal health, you want to keep your waist as small as possible and as close as possible to where it was in your early twenties. If your waist size has increased more than two inches since your early adulthood, it is very likely that you have some excess fat in your belly that is placing you at a higher risk of premature chronic disease.

Here are simple instructions for determining your waist size and relevant waist measurements.

1. Wrap a tape measure around your bare waist, just above your hipbones.

2. Pull the tape measure until it is snug, but not pushing into your skin. Make sure it is level all the way around.

3. Exhale, relax and then take the measurement.

FOR WOMEN	FOR MEN
< 32 inches optimal	< 37 inches optimal
> 35 inches high risk	> 40 inches high risk

The one good thing about belly fat is that it is typically the easiest fat to lose. Because it is so metabolically dynamic and lies in such close proximity to the liver and lots of large blood vessels, the body can more quickly mobilize and burn it.

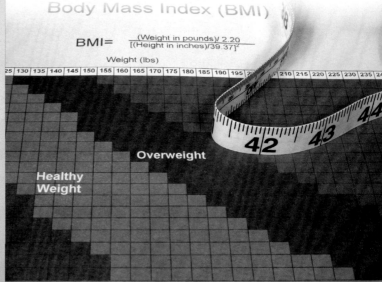

Body Mass Index (BMI)

$$BMI= \frac{(Weight\ in\ pounds)/\ 2.20}{[(Height\ in\ inches)/39.37]^2}$$

Weight (lbs)

...ters for BMI: American Institute for Cancer Research, The National Heart, Lung and Blood Institute, The National Institute of H...

BMI 18.5 to 24.9 kg/m2   BMI 25 to 29.9 kg/m2   BM...

How Much Weight Have You Gained Since Your Early 20s?

Gaining weight in mid-life, regardless of where you start, is bad for your health. Putting on the pounds after your twenties, even if your BMI remains in the normal range, increases your chances of heart disease, type 2 diabetes, colon cancer, uterine cancer, and post-menopausal breast cancer. In other words, even if you were very lean at age 20 (say a BMI of 19) and you are now age 50 and have gained 22 pounds, but still have a BMI in the normal range (say 24)—you are at a substantially higher risk of the aforementioned chronic diseases relative to someone whose weight did not increase throughout their mid-life. I know from talking with lots of people over the years that most are in the dark about the very real dangers of almost any level of adult weight gain.

So here are some stats to give you perspective:

➤ Women who gain more than 20 pounds between the ages of 18 and mid-life double their risk of post-menopausal breast cancer vs. women whose weight remains stable.

➤ Gaining 11 to 18 pounds during adulthood doubles the risk of type 2 diabetes relative to those who have not gained weight.

➤ In two large Harvard-based studies, men and women who put on between 11 and 22 pounds after their early twenties were up to three times more likely to develop heart disease and high blood pressure vs. those who gained five pounds or less.

➤ For every 2-pound increase in weight, the risk of osteoarthritis increases by 9 to 13%.

Unfortunately, mid-life weight gain in America is an almost universal occurrence with less than 10% of the middle age and older adult populations maintaining their weight and waistlines as they were at age 20. In fact, the average American gains about one to two pounds yearly over their adult lifespans. And for most, especially those who have been relatively inactive, they have also lost muscle mass which means that they have actually put on even more fat than is reflected in the scale.

To recap, even very modest weight increases during adulthood significantly increases disease risk and the more you gain the higher your risk. Regardless of where you begin, weight stability over your adult life is central to health maintenance.

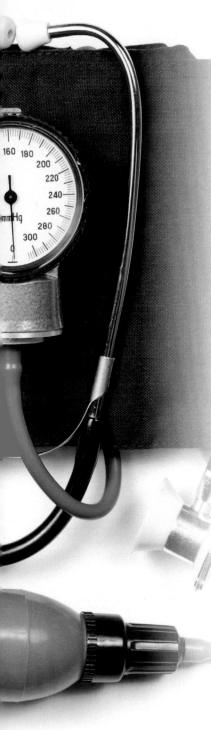

Know Your Metabolic Numbers

Perhaps the single greatest influence excess fat (particularly intra-abdominal fat) has on the body is how it impacts metabolic health. This is of supreme significance to note because your metabolic health transcends all aspects of your health. Simply stated—your metabolism is how your body converts the foods you eat into the energy required to keep your cells, tissues, and organs optimally functioning. Metabolism is the most fundamental of all life processes, and when metabolic dysfunction exists, virtually everything in the body is adversely affected. Indeed, it is the disruption in metabolic function (as a result of carrying too much body fat) that drives the development of many, if not most, of the weight-associated diseases outlined earlier in this chapter.

Hence, it is profoundly helpful, I say essential, to know your "metabolic numbers." Knowing your metabolic metrics provides vital information about your body fat status, especially your belly fat status, and your overall health risk. Here are the key measurements of metabolic function and the ranges that indicate poor vs. optimal metabolic health.

	POOR METABOLIC HEALTH	OPTIMAL METABOLIC
Waist Size	**Females** > 35 inches **Males** > 40 inches	**Females** < 32 inches **Males** < 37 inches
Triglycerides	> 150	< 100
HDL (good) Cholesterol	< 50	60 or higher
Blood Pressure	**Systolic** ≥ 130 **Diastolic** ≥ 85	**Systolic** < 120 **Diastolic** < 80
Fasting Blood Sugar	≥ 110	< 100

Belly Fat = Insulin Resistance = Metabolic Dysfunction

If your metabolic numbers are askew, chances are you are carrying excess body fat, particularly in your mid-section. Even for those of you who appear lean and have a normal BMI, if your metabolic measurements as noted above are out of optimal range, you likely have excess belly blubber that can affect you unfavorably. As discussed earlier in the chapter, belly fat cells secrete chemicals that can incite inflammation throughout the body. These notorious adipokines are so potent that even a small amount of belly fat can be a menace. Unfortunately, one of the most predictable and dire consequences of belly fat-related inflammation is that it interferes with the function and action of the all-important hormone insulin. Insulin is the mother hormone of metabolism and when she cannot do her job properly, the chaotic state that results is called insulin resistance. As would be expected, insulin resistance turns the body into a metabolic train wreck. All aspects of metabolic function become impaired. Fat cells, especially belly fat cells, turn into fat magnets, driving further abdominal weight gain and damaging inflammation—ugh! The body cannot properly process and deliver the fats and sugars that come from the foods you eat to your cells, so fats and sugars begin to accumulate in the wrong places. Sugar (glucose)

> *Over ⅓ of all adult Americans have high (>150) triglycerides. According to the CDC's Diabetes Report Card for 2012, 33% of U.S. adults have prediabetes (fasting blood sugar between 110 and 125), and less than 10% are aware of it.*

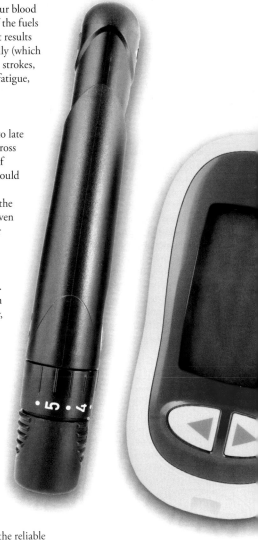

builds up in your blood stream and fats (triglycerides) accrue in your blood stream, muscles, liver, and belly. Because your cells are deprived of the fuels they need to produce energy, they cannot operate effectively. What results from this precarious state of insulin resistance is an even bigger belly (which perpetuates the cycle) and ultimately a higher risk of heart attacks, strokes, metabolic syndrome, type 2 diabetes, future weight gain, obesity, fatigue, sluggish brain function and even some types of cancer.

Belly Fat And Poor Metabolic Health—From Bad To Worse

As in most disease states, there is a spectrum from early and mild to late and severe, and metabolic dysfunction/insulin resistance occurs across this range. Typically, the earliest and the most sensitive indicator of insulin resistance is having an elevated triglyceride level. As you should now understand, elevated triglycerides are also a very reliable and early indicator of excess belly fat. As mentioned earlier, belly fat is the easiest fat to lose and likely why triglycerides are so responsive to even very modest weight loss. In fact, think of your triglycerides as your metabolic and belly fat barometer. The higher your triglycerides, the more belly fat you likely have and the more deranged your metabolism. As more belly fat accumulates, the hormone insulin becomes even more resistant and poor metabolic health progresses. Triglycerides rise even higher, blood pressure trends upward and in the more advanced stages, blood sugar levels increase. In summary, the vicious cycle of metabolic misfortune that results from excess belly fat accumulation goes as follows:

> Belly fat ➤ excess inflammation ➤ insulin resistance ➤ metabolic dysfunction ➤ elevated triglycerides and more belly fat ➤ more inflammation ➤ higher triglycerides/more metabolic dysfunction ➤ elevated blood pressure, low HDL (good cholesterol) and eventually high blood sugar ➤ type 2 diabetes, heart disease, and metabolic syndrome.

As the pathway I outlined illustrates, please make note that blood sugar levels are usually the last metabolic metric to become deranged. In other words, once your fasting blood sugar levels have risen above 110, you have likely had long-standing poor metabolic health. In other words, elevated blood sugar levels should be a HUGE wake up call to take advantage of the reliable strategies and tips in this book to bust your belly fat for good so you can maintain good metabolic health.

The Power Of...
WEIGHT LOSS

In what is perhaps the most stunning confirmation of the goodness of modest weight loss, scientists sought to determine if weight reduction could prevent or delay the onset of type 2 diabetes in high risk study subjects. For this powerful intervention study, 3,234 overweight individuals with pre-diabetes were placed on one of three treatment regimens: diet and lifestyle counseling, the diabetes drug Metformin, or a placebo medication. After 2.8 years, study subjects in the diet and lifestyle group who lost modest amounts of weight (five to seven percent of starting body weight) lowered their risk of developing diabetes by a whopping 58%. It also proved to be much more effective than taking the prescription drug Metformin. The results of this trial were so remarkable that the study was halted a year early to allow those in the placebo group to benefit from the results.

In a recently published update of this landmark study, researchers determined that the benefits of modest weight loss through healthy diet and lifestyle changes remained for up to 10 years, even in the study subjects who gained the weight back at the end of the decade. Now that is encouraging!

Saving The Best News For Last

I have dedicated most of this chapter explaining to you why your body weight matters and how you can reliably assess where you personally stand. I have no doubt that this information is essential for you to know and understand if you aspire to live a long, happy, and productive life. It is my greatest hope however, that this background information will serve to reinforce what I think is the most important general take-away of this entire book—that losing weight, even in modest amounts, can dramatically and decisively improve your health and quality of life. Thankfully there are reams of quality science to back up this wonderful reality. In fact, simply refer back to the long and daunting list of health consequences of excess weight gain on page 14 and imagine the flip side. Need I say more?

The personal power and control you can readily exert over your own health destiny through weight loss and weight control is simply astounding. And when you factor in the improvements in functionality, self-confidence, and general well-being that naturally and very predictably ensue with weight loss, I would hope that everyone would find the prospect of weight control absolutely irresistible.

A Little Loss For Big Gains

Thankfully, one of the most encouraging facts about weight loss is that even modest reductions in body fat can pay huge health dividends. There is convincing data from numerous studies that losing just five to 10% of your current body weight leads to significant improvements in blood sugar, blood pressure, cholesterol levels, and triglyceride levels. For illustration, if you currently weigh 200 pounds and you lose 5% of your body weight (10 pounds), although your weight may remain in the overweight or obese range (190 pounds), you have appreciably lowered your risk of two of our leading killers, cardiovascular disease and type 2 diabetes. And that is worth its weight in gold!

So no matter where you presently are or what your ultimate weight loss goals may be—I hope you will be inspired by the awesome things you can do for your body by losing just a little bit of weight.

Frankly, I remain awed by the radical improvements in health and vitality I have personally witnessed in others through weight loss. In my private wellness practice, individuals seek my dietary and lifestyle counseling on many different fronts and with varying goals. And with rare exception, the common denominator in those who achieve the most sensational and transformative life-enhancing and life-saving results are overweight individuals who lose weight and keep it off by adhering to my guidance.

Which is exactly what lies ahead in this book for you!

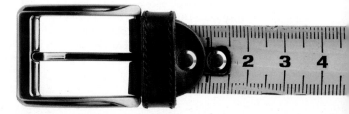

The Weight Of The Matter...

IN SUMMARY

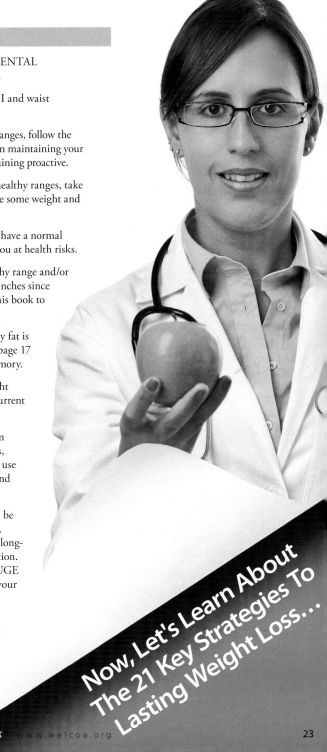

➤ Know that your body weight is of MONUMENTAL importance to your health and quality of life.

➤ Determine your body fat measurements (BMI and waist circumference) as instructed.

➤ If your BMI and waist size are in the normal ranges, follow the guidance in this book to keep them there. Even maintaining your weight living in America takes effort and remaining proactive.

➤ If your BMI and or waist size are not in the healthy ranges, take advantage of the strategies in this book to lose some weight and improve them.

➤ Recognize that you can appear "skinny" and have a normal BMI, yet still have excess belly fat that puts you at health risks.

➤ If your waist measurement is not in the healthy range and/or your waist size has increased more than two inches since your early twenties, follow the guidance in this book to lose weight and reduce your belly fat.

➤ Make sure you understand how and why belly fat is so bad for you. Refer back to the graphic on page 17 as often as needed to cement this in your memory.

➤ Understand that even small amounts of weight gain over your adult life, regardless of your current weight, can increase your health risks.

➤ Know your metabolic numbers as outlined on page 20. If they are not in the optimal ranges, seek the care of your healthcare provider and use the information in this book to lose weight and improve them.

➤ As part of knowing your metabolic numbers, be sure to note that elevated fasting blood sugar, beginning at any level above 100, is a sign of long-standing and more severe metabolic dysfunction. An elevated blood sugar level should be a HUGE wakeup call to take action if you care about your life and your health.

➤ Most importantly, remember that you can wield enormous control over your health and vitality through weight control and that losing even small amounts of weight can change your life and even save your life.

Now, Let's Learn About The 21 Key Strategies To Lasting Weight Loss...

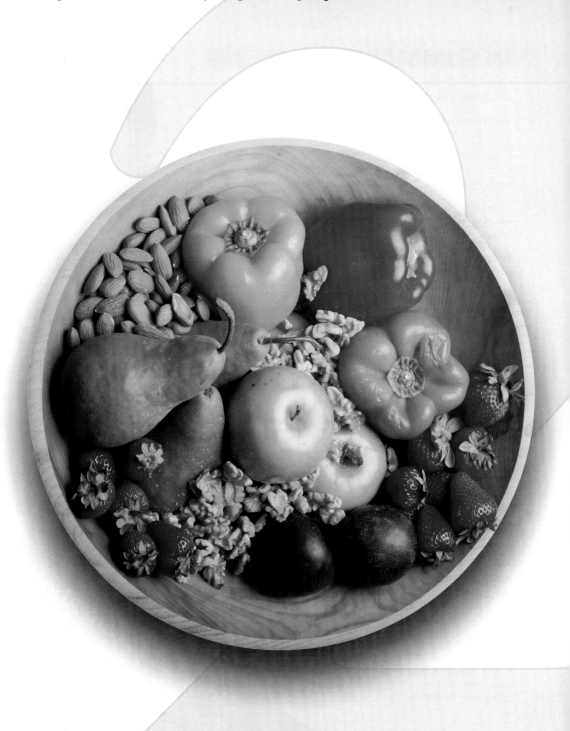

21 Key Strategies To Lasting **Weight Loss**

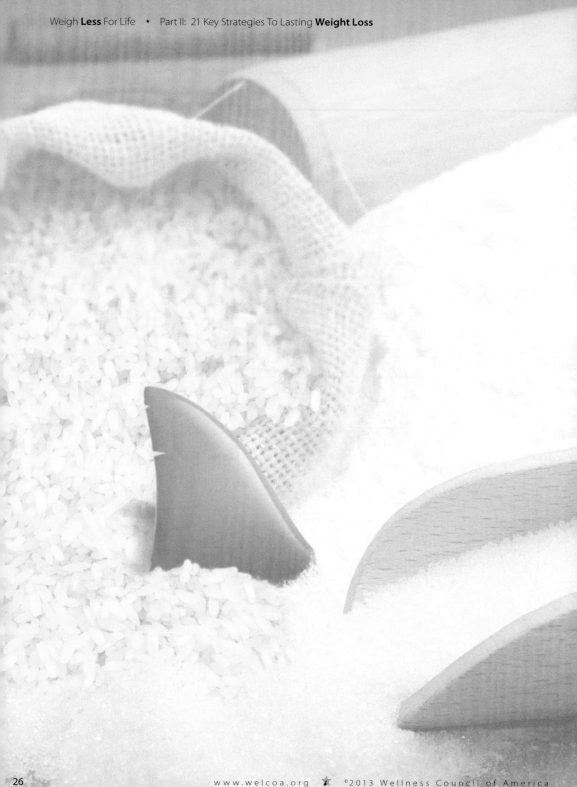

Avoid the
Great White Hazards

Avoid the
Great White Hazards

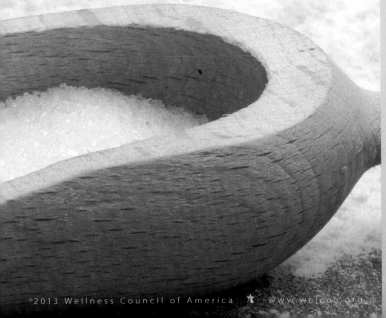

MUCH OF THE BATTLE WITH BODY WEIGHT CAN BE WON SIMPLY BY RIDDING YOUR DIET OF FOODS THAT DRIVE YOUR HUNGER. And the category of food that pops right off the page as the consistent leader in the hunger brigade is what I call "The Great White Hazards." They include: white flour products, white rice, white potatoes, and sugars/sweets.

The root of the appetite-promoting evil of this notorious bunch is their rapid digestibility. Due to their lack of fiber, processed nature, and inherent chemical structure, the "Great White Hazards" are easily and quickly broken down in the digestive tract, giving rise to sudden and large elevations of blood glucose. We refer to quickly digested carbs as "high glycemic load" carbs. Unfortunately, the spikes of blood sugar that ensue when we eat these kinds of carbs are followed shortly thereafter by a precipitous drop in blood sugar. The fallout from this sudden descent in blood glucose is a predictable arousal of appetite. Your brain is keenly sensitive to plummeting blood glucose levels, as it is largely dependent on glucose to provide its enormous energy needs. When blood sugar falls quickly and dips too low, the brain's appetite command center is put on high alert and orders us to go eat. At the same time, the parts of the brain that are involved in putting the brakes on food cravings lose their power.

Unfortunately, the foods we typically crave are more of the "Great White Hazards" because our brains have learned over time that these are the very best foods for swiftly bringing our blood sugar levels back up into the comfort range. The result is a vicious cycle of eating and hunger, and blood sugar peaks and valleys that can incite unhealthy cravings, or even true binging. In fact, recent brain imaging studies in humans have identified specific changes in the brain, in direct response to a drop in blood sugar, that make it extremely difficult to say no to risky, high-calorie foods, especially when you can see them. Overweight individuals appear to be especially vulnerable in this scenario.

The Antidote For Midlife Weight Gain

Midlife weight gain is one of the most predictable and unhealthy accompaniments of aging with most people gaining at least a pound or two a year. Unfortunately midlife comes with a convergence of many different forces that bear on our waistlines, tipping the scales in the positive direction. The six primary drivers of midlife weight gain are:

➤ A slow down in metabolism due to loss of lean body mass (muscle)

➤ A slow down in metabolism due to impaired insulin function (insulin resistance)

➤ More time spent sitting

➤ Less physical activity/exercise

➤ Stress

➤ Inadequate sleep duration or quality

Physical activity reins supreme as the ideal antidote to avoid midlife weight gain because it can improve or alleviate all six of these drivers! (And I do not know of any other factor that can achieve this.) For best results, strive for 30 minutes or more of moderate to vigorous physical activity five or more days a week along with two days of resistance (weight-bearing) exercise each week.

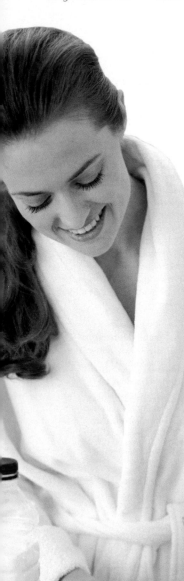

Dr. Ann's...
PLAN OF ACTION

Luckily, ridding your diet of the "Great White Hazards" is a very straightforward and truly life changing step in the right direction. Here are my directives for triumph:

➤ Restrict all white flour products, white rice, white potatoes, and sweets. White flour products are everywhere and include: white breads, bagels, biscuits, rolls, crackers, pancakes, waffles, dumplings, pretzels, and pizza dough.

➤ Always choose the fiber and nutrient-rich carbs as a totally healthy and filling alternative—fruits, vegetables, physically intact whole grains, and beans. These carbs are fantastic for appetite control because they have a much lower glycemic load. Meaning they will not drive your blood sugar levels up high and quickly.

➤ Good choices for physically intact whole grains are oatmeal, brown or black rice, quinoa, barley, farro, and bulgur.

➤ Enjoy sweet potatoes over white potatoes.

➤ Choose multigrain or whole wheat pasta over traditional white pasta.

➤ Other wholesome starch options to replace the processed white ones are winter squashes, any variety of beans, lentils, and peas.

➤ Strictly avoid any sugar-fortified beverages, such as sodas and fruit drinks, and sugary breakfast cereals. These hazards are the very worst offenders for driving blood sugar levels down too low too fast.

➤ For dessert, have a prudent portion of high-quality dark chocolate (see pages 54–59).

➤ For additional motivation, keep in mind that the "Great White Hazards" have also been linked with a number of our leading killers, including heart disease, type 2 diabetes, metabolic syndrome, and some cancers. Also be encouraged by the fact that your taste buds will change as you shift to nature-made vs. factory-made refined carbs—you will tend to crave the good in lieu of the bad.

RESEARCH CORNER

Great White Hazards Make Us Eat More

A recent study at Harvard University showed just how influential the glycemic response of various carbs could be in determining how much we eat. In the study, researchers fed 12 obese teenage boys identical breakfast and lunch meals on three separate occasions. The two identical breakfast and lunch test meals were high, medium, or low glycemic.

The high glycemic meal consisted of sweetened, instant oatmeal, the medium glycemic meal was steel-cut oatmeal, and the low glycemic meal was a vegetable omelet served with fruit.

Despite the fact that all three test-meals had an identical number of calories, the study subjects ate 81% more calories after the high glycemic breakfasts and lunches, and 51% more calories after the medium glycemic meals, when compared to the low glycemic meals.

The investigators also measured the study subject's blood glucose levels. They were able to clearly document that the rapid rise in blood glucose levels after the high glycemic meals induced a cascade of metabolic changes that promoted appetite and increased subsequent food intake.

Low Glycemic Meals Help Us Eat Less

Scientists consistently observe that eating meals with a low glycemic load stifles appetite. To further elucidate the science behind these findings, researchers at King's College London evaluated the effects of a single low vs. high glycemic meal on gut hormones involved in appetite control. In a group of 12 healthy study subjects, the scientists found that blood levels of the potent appetite-quieting hormone GLP-1 were 20% higher after the low glycemic meal vs. the high glycemic meal. The investigators concluded that their results provide a physiologic mechanism to clarify how low glycemic foods help us eat less.

In a powerful landmark report that sought to drill down to what specific dietary and lifestyle factors most closely correlated to weight gain over time, Harvard researchers uncovered some very striking and consistent findings. This behemoth of a study involved over 115,000 adults followed for up to 20 years. Of all the factors they followed including diet, exercise, sleep, and TV viewing, food choices were the most influential. The specific foods associated with the greatest weight gain over time were (in descending order): potato chips, other forms of white potatoes, sugary beverages, unprocessed meats, and processed meats. Thankfully, the researchers also found that increasing the consumption of certain foods protected against weight gain. These "eat more–weigh less" foods were (in descending order) yogurt, nuts, fruits, whole grains, and vegetables.

In summary, the most effective strategies for avoiding long term weight gain included:

> Doing your carbs right! Avoiding the great white hazards—white flour products, white rice, white potatoes, and sugar (especially sugary beverages). Eating more fruits, veggies, and whole grains.

> Eating nuts and yogurt (I say plain) regularly.

> Restricting meats, including the processed varieties.

Four Ways To Make Your Pasta Dishes Healthier

Pasta can fit deliciously into optimal appetite control, especially if you follow these four guidelines.

1 Choose "multigrain", whole wheat, brown rice, or soba (buckwheat) pastas over conventional white pasta. I love the Barilla Plus brand of multigrain pasta. Its taste and texture is just like regular pasta—try it!

2 Cook it al dente (a slightly chewy texture). This will reduce its glycemic response, which is better for your arteries and your metabolism.

3 Flavor it with a little extra virgin olive oil and lemon, or a tomato-based sauce instead of cream or cheese-based Alfredo-type sauces.

4 Combine your pasta with a variety of vegetables and herbs to give it color, flavor, hunger-quieting oomph and to give YOU life!

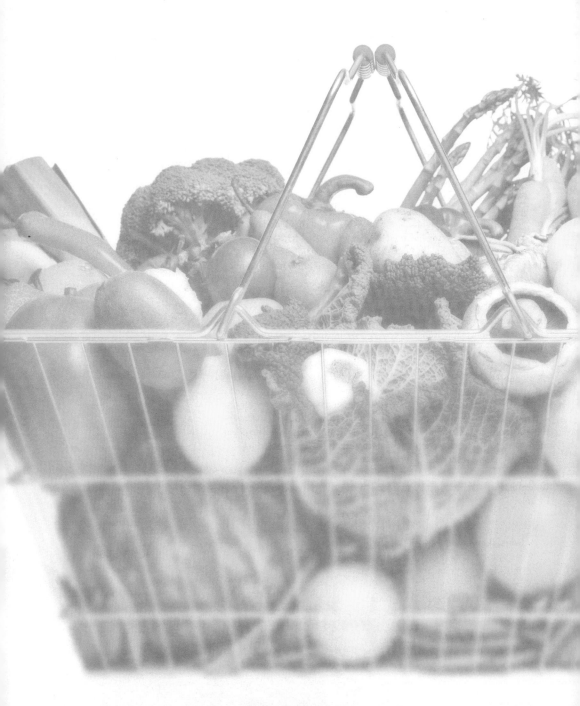

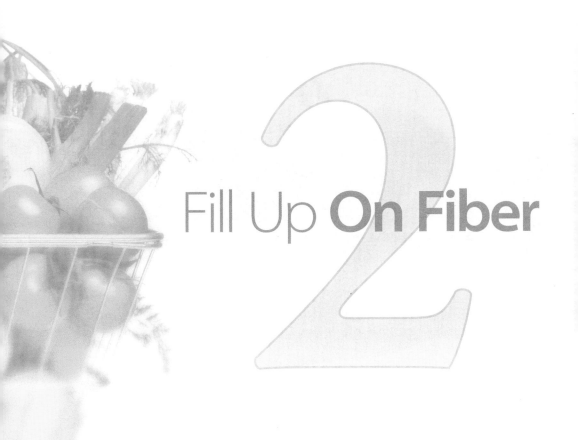

Fill Up **On Fiber**

Fill Up
On Fiber
2

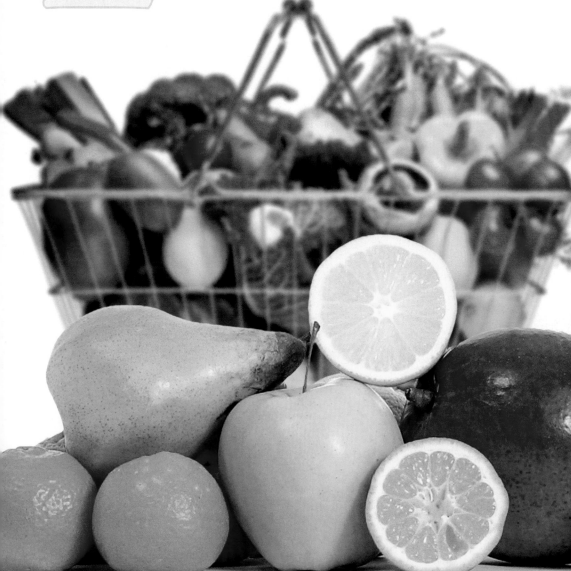

DIETARY FIBER HAS A WELL-DESERVED AND SPARKLING REPUTATION AS A KEY DEFENSE AGAINST OUR MOST DREADED CHRONIC DISEASES, BUT FIGHTING FAT IS ARGUABLY WHERE IT SHINES MOST BRILLIANTLY. I consider dietary fiber the "secret weapon" for weight and appetite control.

One of the most predictable and defining features in the diets of people who achieve long-term success with body weight is their abundant intake of fiber-rich foods. And it is no wonder. Fiber offers a multitude of slimming features. Through its volume and physical bulking abilities, fiber effectively "fills" your stomach up while providing zero calories. This simple property of fiber is invaluable for hunger management because when it comes to satisfying the human appetite, volume trumps calories. This means that the body's desire for a given volume of food supersedes its calorie demands for appetite control.

In addition to providing a physical sense of fullness in your tummy, fiber's "volumizing" effects can also augment the release of appetite-suppressing hormones from the gastrointestinal tract. This means less hunger faster. As a final bonus, fiber can also slow the digestive process. This has two fringe benefits. First, food will ultimately stay in your stomach for a longer period of time, which means you will feel satisfied longer. And second, because fiber hinders digestion, it will naturally soften the peaks and valleys of blood glucose fluctuations that can awaken and incite the inner cookie monster.

Tragically, despite fiber's awesome benefits for health and body weight, we are running a huge fiber deficit in this country. The average American diet is painfully deficient in this natural appetite suppressant. Current intakes hover around a paltry 12 grams daily. For optimal health and appetite control, the body requires at least 14 grams for every 1,000 calories consumed. This translates to a minimum of about 25 grams daily for women and 30 grams daily for men. For a big dose of aspiration, consider that our ancient ancestors likely consumed around 150 grams a day! I am not going to let the cave men show me up.

Busting Belly Fat

There is now a mountain of scientific evidence that belly (visceral) fat is particularly dangerous so I am excited to share results from a new report that identified two simple strategies for fighting this menace. For this evaluation, Wake Forest researchers followed 1,114 people over a five-year period to determine what dietary and lifestyle factors may reduce belly fat accumulation. Thankfully, the researchers found that both soluble fiber and moderate physical activity proved to be winning waist-whittling endeavors. For every 10 grams of soluble fiber consumed daily, belly fat was reduced by 3.7%. Moderate physical activity (like brisk walking) proved to be an even better belly fat buster—slowing the build up of belly fat by 7.4%.

So you can just say whoa to belly fat! Be sure to engage in at least 30 minutes of moderate physical activity daily (the more, the better!) and eat an abundance of foods high in soluble fiber. Here are your best food choices: beans (any variety), peas, barley, flax seeds, chia seeds, oats, oat bran, avocado, carrots, collards, oranges and apples.

Rein In Your Appetite

It is well established that external visuals of high-calorie foods can drive us to desire them and seek them out, especially when we are hungry. Here are some simple strategies to help you avoid this high-risk situation:

1 Do not leave your home hungry. Our external environments are filled with alluring visuals of high risk, bad-for-you foods. Think billboards, fast food signage, etc.

2 Do not go to the grocery store hungry. Here you will encounter the real thing—not just the pictures!

3 If you bring high-risk foods into your home (which I do not recommend), keep them out of sight. Even within the refrigerator or cupboard it is helpful to hide them behind more healthy foods. Remember—"out of sight out of mind"—so cover the ice cream up with bags of frozen spinach.

4 If traveling by air—watch those airports! Actually, do not watch those airports. Put up blinders as you walk through the concourse (do not look at the Cinnabon counter or the Haagen Daaz counter!) And always pack healthy, travel-friendly snacks to avoid ravenous hunger in the toxic nutritional environments of airports. I travel frequently on business and my favorite snacks to pack are nuts, dark chocolate, whole fresh fruits, soy nuts, and dried wasabi peas.

Dr. Ann's...
PLAN OF ACTION

To get more fiber in your daily diet, focus on eating the following foods often and in abundance:

➤ **Beans:** Measure for measure, beans provide more fiber than any other food. A single ½ cup serving dishes up 6 plus grams. Enjoy any variety in any form—canned, fresh, frozen, or dried.

➤ **Fruits And Vegetables:** Berries, apples, sweet peas, canned tomato products, canned pumpkin, cauliflower, avocados, spinach, asparagus, broccoli, carrots, Brussels sprouts, sweet potatoes, okra, and winter squash are the fiber superstars.

➤ **High-Fiber Whole-Grain Cereals:** Choose those with at least five grams of fiber per serving.

➤ **Physically Intact Whole Grains:** Oatmeal, brown rice, quinoa, barley, bulgur, etc.

Please note that isolated fiber artificially added (typically labeled as inulin, chicory root, oat fiber, wheat fiber, or maltodextrin) to processed foods like breads, cereals, and meal replacement bars has not been shown to provide the benefits of fiber that is naturally a part of whole foods like those noted above.

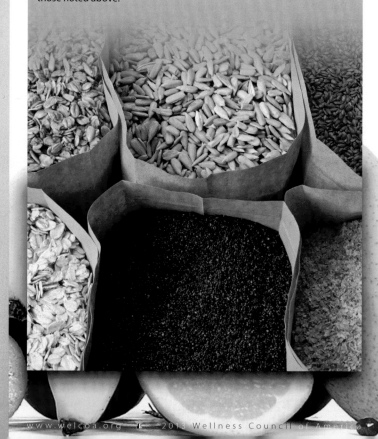

RESEARCH CORNER

The Skinny On Fiber

Fiber's effect on fullness has been put to the test in several scientific studies. Here are two notable ones.

To test the impact of dietary fiber on feelings of fullness and blood levels of the appetite-suppressing hormone CCK, researchers at the University of California-Davis fed an equal group of men and women three different breakfast meals varying in fiber and fat content. The test meals were low-fiber, low-fat; low-fiber, high-fat; or high-fiber, low-fat.

Both groups reported greater fullness with the high-fiber meals, and in the women, blood levels of CCK were significantly higher in the high-fiber, low-fat meal vs. the low-fat, low-fiber meal. Investigators concluded that fiber appears to aid in appetite suppression by contributing to a greater volume of food in the GI tract and boosting the release of the appetite-suppressive hormone CCK.

In a large Harvard based study, researchers followed the dietary fiber intake of 74,000 women participating in the Nurse's Health Study. Over the 12-year study period, women who consumed the most dietary fiber had a 49% lower risk of significant weight gain than those consuming the least.

> *One of the most predictable and defining features in the diets of people who achieve long-term success with body weight is their abundant intake of fiber-rich foods.*

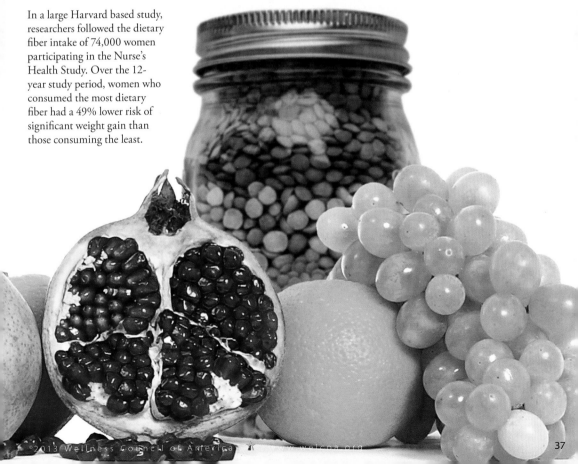

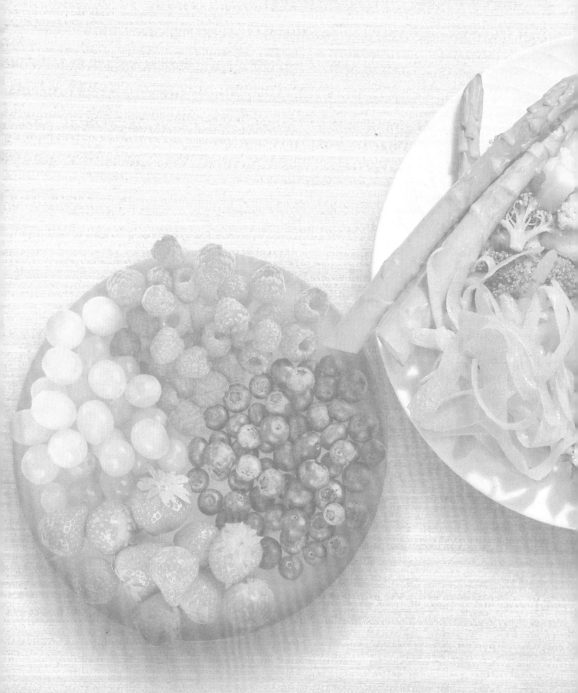

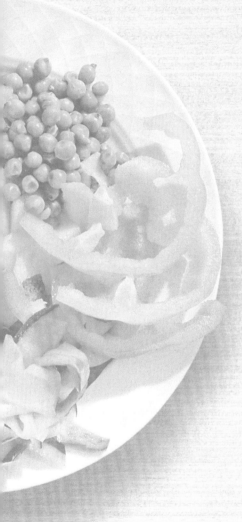

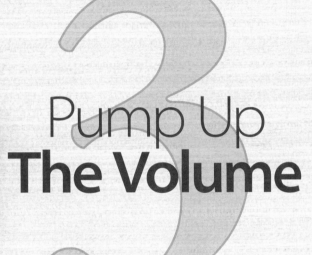

Pump Up
The Volume

Pump Up The
Volume

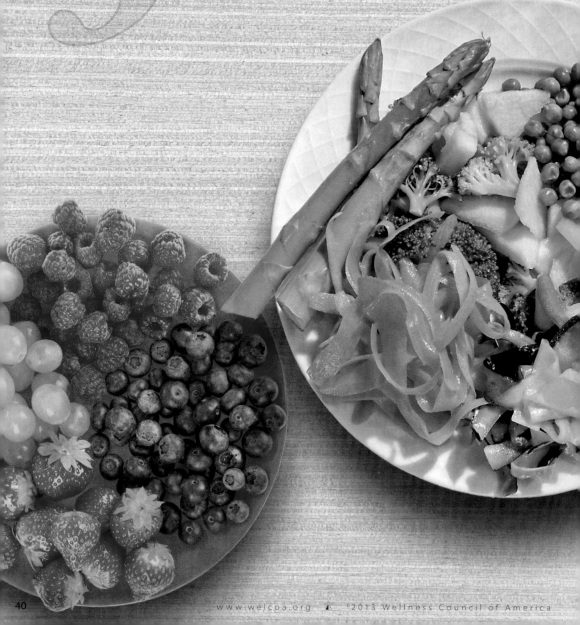

WHEN IT COMES TO EATING LESS, IT REALLY BOILS DOWN TO QUANTITY... AND QUALITY. If you make a consistent effort to load up on high-volume foods that are low in calories, you won't have room for the other junk that often ruins your best weight loss intentions.

When it comes to what high-volume, low-calorie foods to choose, far and away your best choices are the "big yet skinny" fruits and non-starchy vegetables. These slimming foods are low in calories and big in volume because they have so much water and fiber. This unique fruit and veggie feature is oh-so-valuable in the quest to eat less because volume trumps calories when it comes to satisfying the desire for food.

Research has consistently shown that filling your stomach with a certain volume of food can shut off the brain's appetite center, regardless of how many calories come along with it. In fact, it appears that our bodies desire a given volume of food first and foremost over a certain number of calories.

This reality is instrumental for manipulating hunger and appetite. And in addition to quelling hunger, eating large quantities of fruits and veggies can also diminish the sense of deprivation people feel when they try to lose weight. Let's face it—we like to eat and we like to eat lots, and thankfully with fruits and veggies we can be glutinous without the risks. Even the sight of a plate filled with food—in this case fruits and vegetables, automatically makes you feel more satisfied! Considering all of this produce oomph, you should make it your goal to look for every possible opportunity to "bulk up" your meals and dishes with as many hefty, yet low-calorie fruits and vegetables as possible.

Let me give you a simple example to make this point: If you ate a big plate piled high with steamed broccoli, you would feel satisfied (likely even stuffed) from its volume, yet have only consumed about 130 calories. This eat less strategy has been shown to be highly effective in studies. When it comes to fruits and veggies, eating more and weighing less is real! And of course this eat less directive also taps into the extraordinary capacity of fruits and veggies to boost overall vitality. Bottom line—eating fruits and veggies comes with a built-in guarantee—the more you eat them, the healthier and the leaner you will be!

The Fat That's "Most Filling"

In a fascinating report that sought to investigate how various natural fats affect satiety (the feeling of fullness), olive oil came out on top. For three months researchers had study subjects supplement their normal daily diets with 500 grams of low-fat yogurt spiked with one of four fats—lard, butter fat, rapeseed oil, or olive oil.

Those consuming the olive oil yogurt had the highest levels of the satiety hormone serotonin in their blood and also reported the yogurt to be "very filling." The researchers then dug a little deeper to determine what aspects of the olive oil could be responsible for its superior hunger-quieting effects. Two chemicals unique to olive oil's aroma extracts were found to be the likely active ingredients. They worked by maintaining the level of glucose in the bloodstream which helps keep the brain's hunger center in the off position longer. Relative to olive oils from Spain, Greece, and Australia—Italian olive oil provided the greatest concentrations of these appetite-suppressive aroma compounds.

Dr. Ann's...
PLAN OF ACTION

Eating less with more fruits and vegetables is not only healthy; it can be life changing and delicious, too! Just follow these simple steps to success.

➤ "Volumize" your meals and snacks with as many high-fiber, high-water fruits and vegetables as possible. The best choices include the following:

- **Fruits**—berries, cherries, plums, any whole citrus fruits, melon, grapes, peaches, apples, pears, and kiwi. Avoid "low-volume" dried fruits.
- **Vegetables**—cabbage, kale, broccoli, cauliflower, Brussels sprouts, collards, carrots, garlic, onions, leeks, celery, cucumbers, tomatoes, asparagus, spinach, dark lettuces, bell peppers, and mushrooms.

➤ "Double up" your fruit and vegetable side dishes.

➤ Always go for non-starchy vegetable sides in lieu of starchy white carbs like white potatoes, pasta, and white rice.

➤ Feature vegetables as the star ingredients in your main dishes.

➤ Fill at least ½ of your plate up with veggies before dishing up the rest of your meal.

➤ If veggies are called for in recipes, add in extra. If they are not called for, add them anyway or look for a recipe that does. Dishes like salads, soups, and stews are especially accommodating to produce.

➤ Snack on raw fruits and vegetables.

➤ If you are not already a veggie lover, try roasting your vegetables. Roasting naturally brings out the flavor and natural sweetness in vegetables, which makes them delectable. I have several free recipes on my website: **www.DrAnnWellness.com**.

➤ Strive to always begin your meals by eating any fruits and veggies on the plate first. We tend to eat the most of what we start with, and starting with veggies has been shown to help you eat less of the other foods on your plate.

↙ RESEARCH CORNER

"Volumizing" With Vegetables

Filling up on fruits and vegetables is one of the most powerful pathways to help you eat less. In one weight loss study, obese study subjects who had the greatest reduction in energy density over the six month study period, i.e., those who ate the most fruits and veggies, lost more than two times as much weight as those with the least reduction in energy density. What's more—the fruit and veggie eaters literally ate ¾ of a pound more food a day! As a double bonus, including more fruits and veggies in your diet not only reduces caloric intake, but also dramatically boosts the nutritional quality of your diet. I always include at least one cup of fruit at breakfast and 1½ cups of veggies at lunch and dinner. If you have not already achieved this milestone in healthy living, I urge you to do so. I know of no other nutritional undertaking that will more quickly transform the way you look and feel, while simultaneously turning you into a biological bastion.

Dr. Ann's List Of Superstar Foods For Appetite Control

➤ Lean animal proteins— fish, shellfish, skinless poultry, omega-3 eggs, low-fat dairy products (especially plain Greek yogurt).

➤ Plant proteins—whole soy foods, nuts, seeds, and beans (especially beans!).

➤ Non-starchy veggies— cabbage, kale, broccoli, cauliflower, Brussels sprouts, collards, carrots, onions, leeks, tomatoes, asparagus, spinach, dark lettuces, bell peppers, avocados.

➤ Mushrooms.

➤ Non-tropical fruits— berries, cherries, plums, apples, pears, grapes, kiwi, peaches, and melon.

➤ Physically intact whole grains—oats, brown or black rice, barley, bulgur, quinoa, kasha, farro, etc.

➤ High fiber cereals— choose those with at least five grams of fiber per serving (avoid those with >10 grams of sugar).

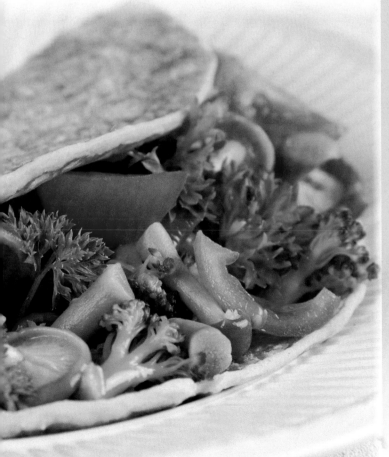

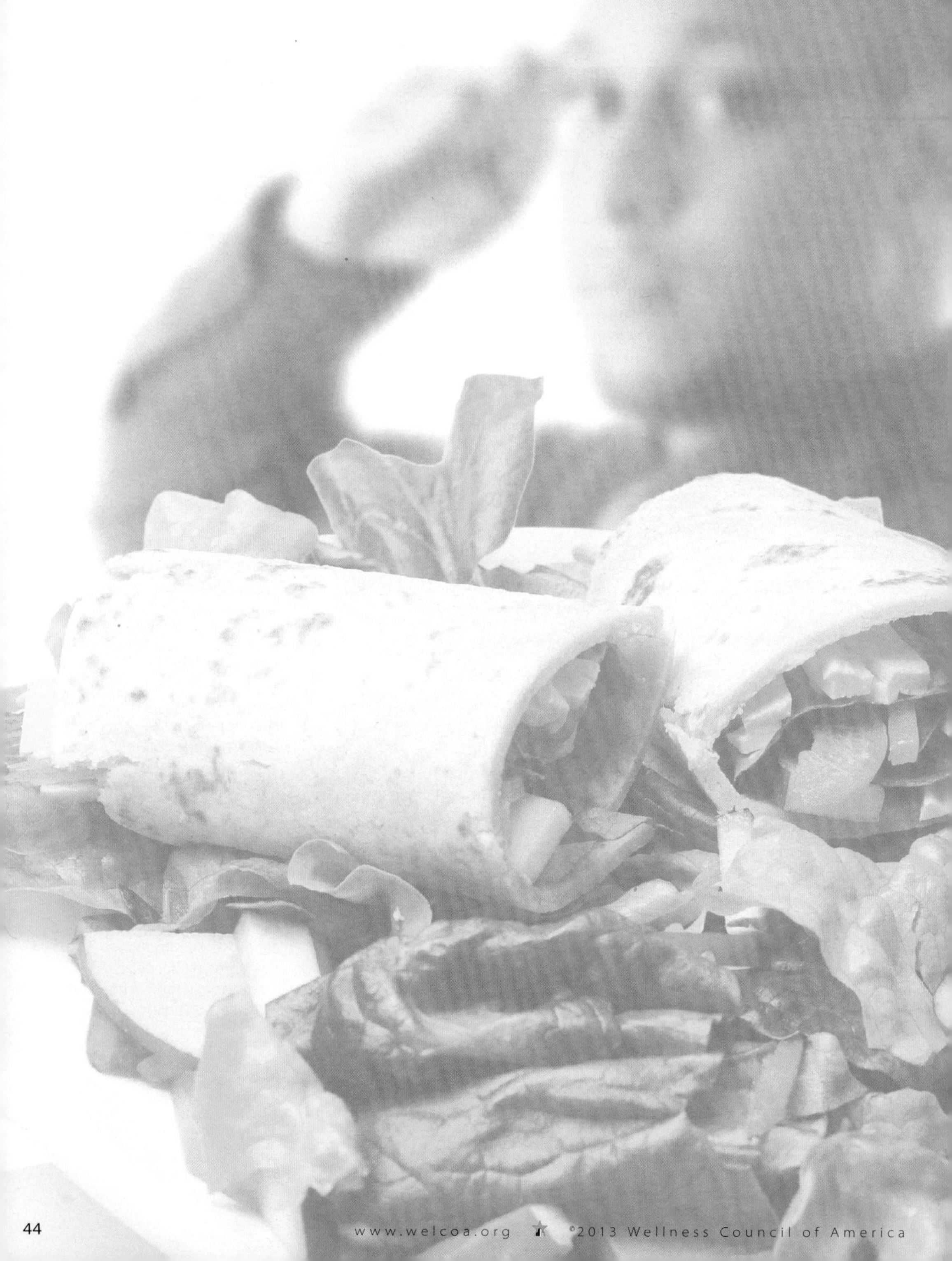

Give Your Plate
Your Full Attention

Give Your Plate
Your Full
Attention

OF ALL THE QUICK AND EASY THINGS WE CAN DO TO HELP OURSELVES EAT LESS, SIMPLY PAYING ATTENTION MAY BE THE MOST POWERFUL AND EFFECTIVE. An intriguing and growing body of impressive science is showing that the more attentive and mindful we can be as we eat, the less we eat now AND later. Meaning, if we can give the foods we are eating during a meal or snack our full, undivided attention and awareness, we tend to eat less calories during that eating occasion and during the next feeding. For example, if you eat your breakfast while distracted as you watch TV or drive to work, you are more apt to consume excess calories during that breakfast and during the subsequent lunch. In fact, studies show that the influences of distraction during eating have an even greater impact on over-consumption of calories at the subsequent feeding. Yes, eating mindlessly encourages overeating in the present and in the future, so be aware of that!

Scientist now recognize that the cognitive (brain-based) processes of attention and memory have a strong influence on appetite and how much we eat. To put it in simple terms—the more aware we are while eating, the less likely we are to over-consume. Additionally, being more attentive during eating enhances memory of the foods consumed, which helps us eat less food later on.

> *Aside from curbing your food intake, eating mindfully has several other fantastic fringe benefits that you can look forward to. These include enhancing the pleasure and enjoyment of eating, helping us discern between emotional hunger (a powerful stimulus for overeating) and real hunger, developing a more positive relationship with food, and reducing stress.*

When You Eat... MATTERS

Most everyone already knows that what and how much you eat matters for weight loss. But there is growing evidence that when you eat matters too. In the very first large scale study of its type, investigators sought to examine how "meal timing" affects weight loss.

Specifically, researchers followed 420 overweight study subjects who were placed on a 20-week weight loss program. The study subjects were divided in two equal groups and instructed to consume equal calories, but with different timings for the main meal, in this case lunch. "Early-eaters" consumed lunch before 3PM, and "late-eaters" consumed lunch after 3 pm. Relative to the early-eaters, the late-eaters lost significantly less weight, lost weight more slowly, and exhibited less insulin sensitivity (a risk factor for type 2 diabetes). The late eaters were also more likely to skip breakfast and consume less food at breakfast.

The researchers concluded that the timing of large meals could be an important factor in weight loss success. Based on the studies I have reviewed, I highly recommend that you strive to eat most of your calories in the earlier parts of the day and go lighter on dinner.

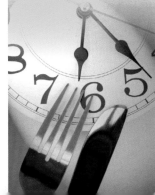

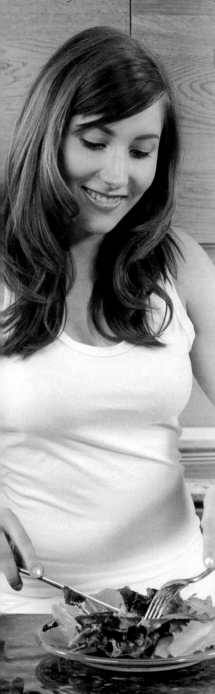

Dr. Ann's...

PLAN OF ACTION

To fully leverage the power of attentive eating to help you consume less, here are my best tips for developing mindfulness during mealtimes.

➤ Reserve eating just for eating. Never engage in other distracting activities during meal or snack times. Avoid watching TV, listening to radio commentary, driving a car, reading, writing, texting, answering emails etc. Engaging in conversation with dining partners should be the only competing activity during your eating occasions.

➤ Sit down to eat your meals—preferably at a set table. Strictly avoid eating directly out of a food package, box, or bag.

➤ Before you begin to eat, take a few seconds to calm and center your body and mind. Strive to let go of any negative emotions. Make note of your current hunger and where it ranges on the scale from minimal hunger to ravenous hunger.

➤ Recall what you ate at your previous meal. If you can remember it as very satisfying that is a bonus.

➤ Be conscious of portions control. For best results, limit what you will be eating to what fits into your own two hands cupped together minus any fruits and veggies (no need to limit these bulky weigh less foods).

➤ Carefully and with your full attention look at all of your food before you begin to eat.

➤ Eat with a positive and joyful attitude. Acknowledge that foods are important for nourishment and health, but also for pleasure and comfort.

➤ With each bite of food, pay close attention to the food leaving your plate and entering your mouth. Make note with all of your senses to its appearance, taste, aroma, and texture. As eating progresses, be aware of your hunger mitigating. Stop eating when you feel full.

➤ Leave any visual evidence of foods consumed on your plate—food wrappers, shells from nuts or shellfish, bones from meat or fish, corn cobs, inedible seeds, etc.

➤ Never go back for seconds for at least 20 minutes after your first bite of food.

➤ When you're done eating, make a mental note that you are comfortably sated (full), and get up from the table or, at a minimum, push your dinnerware away from your place at the table or request that it be removed.

The studies conducted to evaluate mindless vs. attentive eating have identified four effective approaches to help us eat with greater attentiveness, with the goal of eating less. They include:

1. Eating without the presence of distracting stimuli, with particular attention to AVOIDING watching television during eating.

2. Specifically recalling in your mind all of the foods eaten at the previous snack or meal just before you begin to eat the following meal. Even better, recall the foods and "remember" them as satisfying.

3. Being purposely aware and in the moment throughout the entire eating episode.

4. Paying attention with all of your senses (sight, smell, taste, touch, and sound) as you eat to strengthen memory of the foods consumed.

Aside from curbing your food intake, eating mindfully has several other fantastic fringe benefits that you can look forward to. These include enhancing the pleasure and enjoyment of eating, helping discern between emotional hunger (a powerful stimulus for overeating) and real hunger, developing a more positive relationship with food, and reducing stress. Perhaps the very best effect from cultivating mindfulness as you eat is greater happiness. We are almost always happier when our minds are in the moment than when they are wandering elsewhere. In summary, mindful eating pays deliciously promising dividends both on the scale and in your quality of life.

Research CORNER

Pay Attention To Eat Less Now And Later

In a compelling review of 24 former studies that focused on eating while distracted vs. eating while attentive—the results were noteworthy. The more distracted and the less mindful we are during eating, the more we tend to eat in that sitting, and even more so, during the next feeding. For this evaluation, scientists selected tightly controlled intervention studies that monitored how study participant's attention, memory, and awareness of eating influenced how much they ate. On average, consuming food while distracted, like watching TV increased the amount of food eaten by 10%. Even more notable, eating with distractions increased what study subjects ate at the subsequent meal by more than 25%. Study interventions that enhanced memories of the foods eaten at previous meals decreased the amount consumed at the following meals by 10%. Taken together, these results indicate that distracted, mindless eating can boost what we eat by as much as 50%!

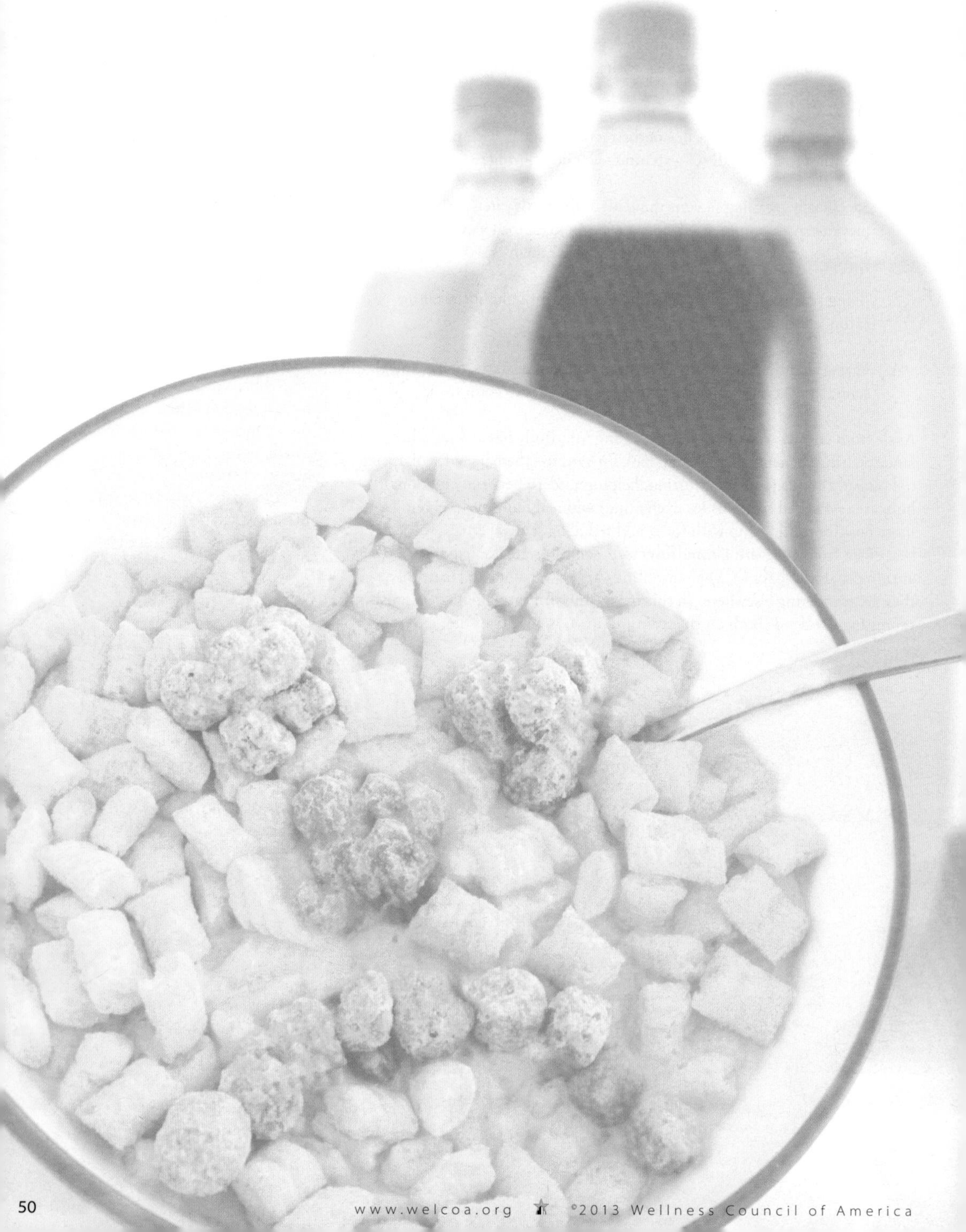

Restrict Your
Intake Of Fructose

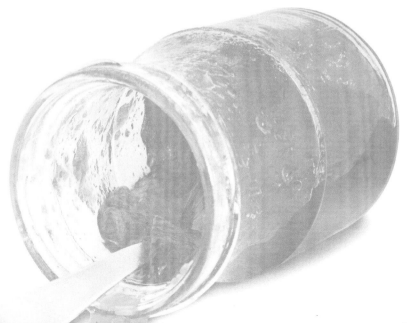

Restrict Your
Intake Of Fructose

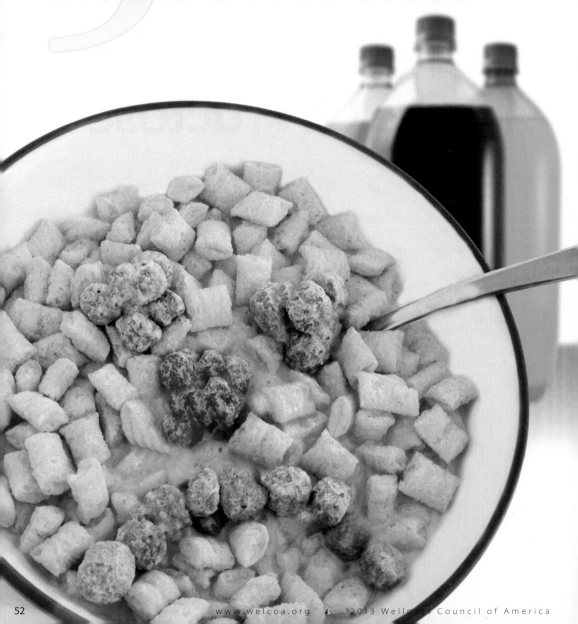

OF ALL THE DIETARY CULPRITS THAT UNDERLIE OUR CURRENT OBESITY CRISIS, PERHAPS NONE IS SINGLED OUT MORE OFTEN THAN FRUCTOSE. Indeed, there is a dead-on, steep and precipitous parallel between our burgeoning waistlines and our enormous intakes of this simple sugar. We are currently consuming record amounts of fructose with the lion's share coming from sugary beverages and sweets. And it certainly appears that this fructose free-for-all really is fueling and feeding our bulging bellies. Indeed, riveting new research has shown that fructose, through all sorts of metabolic mischief, is uniquely fattening. This stealth fat builder is particularly dicey for appetite control. Unlike its simple-sugar counterpart glucose, fructose does not stimulate the release of insulin or leptin, two key hormones integral to quieting our hunger. Even more alarming, recent laboratory studies have indicated that the metabolism of fructose in the brain can actually increase food intake by stimulating the appetite center.

Unfortunately, fructose currently makes up about 12–15% of all the calories consumed in America, constituting a four-fold increase from 30 years ago. For optimal health, experts recommend that fructose comprise no more than three percent of total calories. In addition to obesity and weight gain, dietary fructose has also been implicated as a big driver of many other now epidemic conditions including: metabolic syndrome, type 2 diabetes, kidney disease, elevated triglycerides, and fatty liver disease.

Dr. Ann's...
PLAN OF ACTION

Bringing your fructose intake down to more acceptable levels is essential for achieving a healthy weight and protecting your overall health. Here is my best advice.

➤ Strictly avoid all sugary beverages—sodas, fruits drinks, fruit juice, energy drinks, sweet tea, and dessert cof-fees. Liquid forms of fructose are especially high risk.

➤ Limit your intake of dessert foods and sweets. Choose a prudent portion of dark chocolate instead (See pages 54–59).

➤ Steer clear of sugary cereals. Choose those with less than 10 grams of sugar per serving.

➤ Be aware of the processed foods that frequently come with significant amounts added fructose—fat-free salad dressings, fruit-flavored yogurts, some breads, jelly, and prepared tomato sauces.

Research
CORNER

The Findings On Fructose

A recent animal study provides alarming evidence about the effects of a high-fructose diet. Researchers fed laboratory rats two diets with the same number of calories, but differing in fructose content. One group ate a 60% fructose diet, while the control group was fed a fructose-free diet.

After six months, half of the rats in each group were switched to a two-week high-fat diet. Rats who had consumed the high-fructose diet prior to switching to the new diet gained significantly more weight when compared to the control group. Additionally, the investigators were able to show that the fructose-fed rats became leptin "resistant," which means that they lost the powerful appetite-suppressive effects that leptin normally induces.

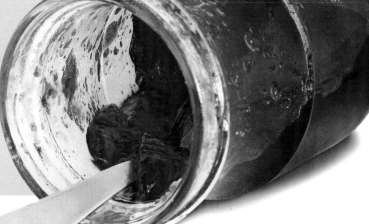

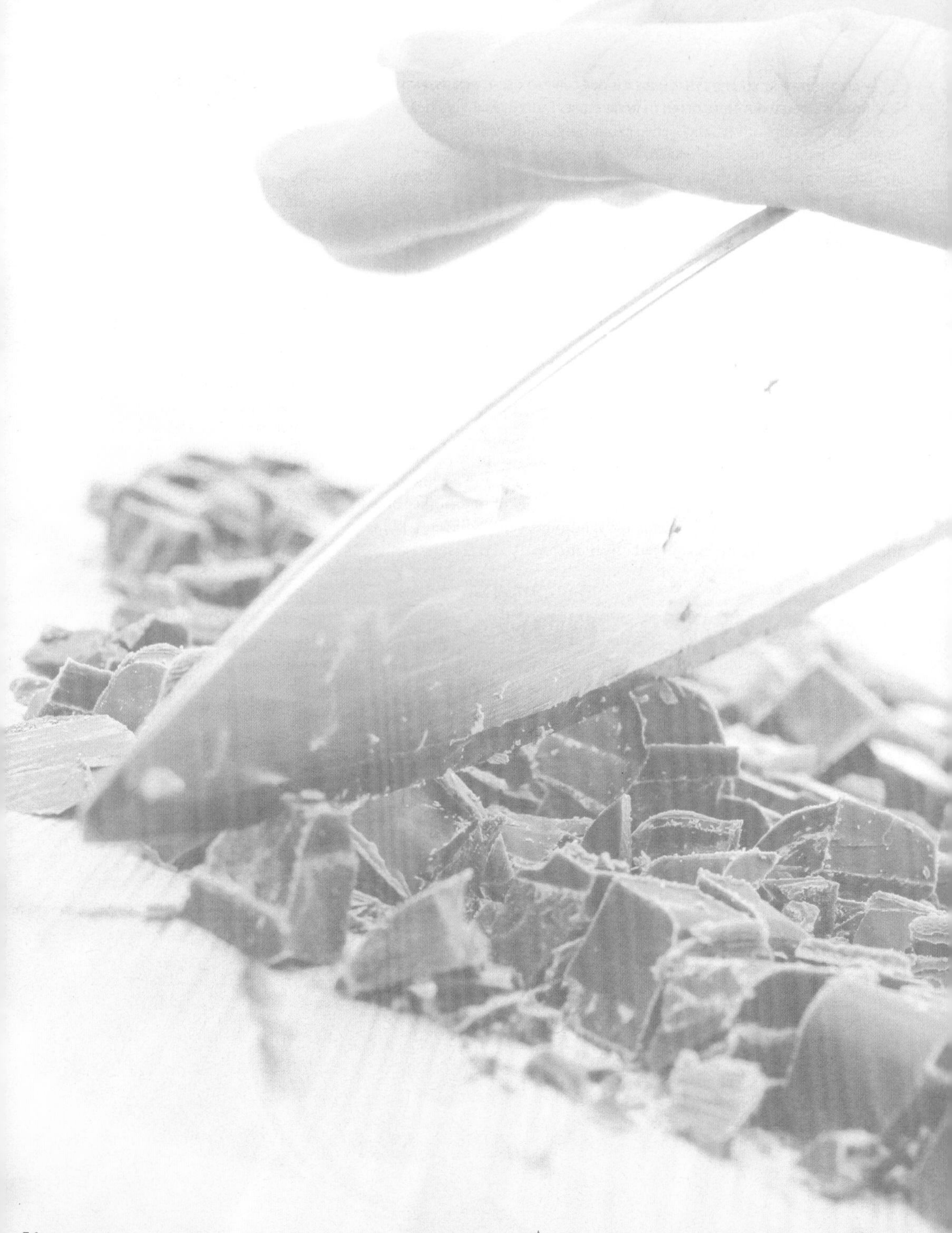

Indulge In
Dark Chocolate

Indulge In
Dark Chocolate

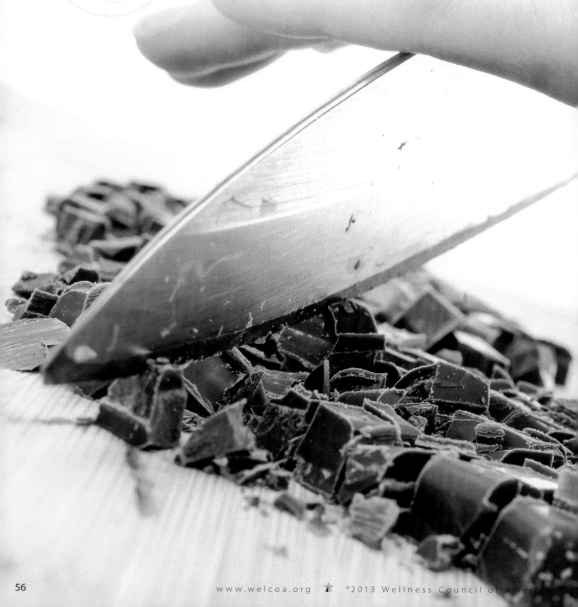

I F THERE'S ONE THING THAT ALMOST ALL OF US HAVE IN COMMON, IT'S A SWEET TOOTH. And because life is for living, it would be unrealistic to expect any of us to completely forgo sweets.

Thankfully, recent research is indicating that you don't have to. There is a sweet that you can enjoy without fear—dark chocolate.

This delectable, truly healthy treat has been rocketed to the forefront over the past few years by scoring one scientific victory after another. Its accomplishments include boosting brainpower, lifting mood, and improving cardiovascular health, among others.

Intriguing research shows that as "sweets" go, dark chocolate may be particularly adept at shutting off that sweet tooth by providing a greater feeling of satisfaction and satiety than other sweets. Researchers speculate that dark chocolate's potent "bittersweet" taste conveys stronger and more intense signals from the taste buds in the mouth to the satiety center of the brain.

For many, this same intense flavor also means that less chocolate can do the trick. The rich and robust flavor of dark chocolate lingers in your mouth a bit longer. Additionally, the bit of fat in dark chocolate provides quick appetite suppression and can also hinder the absorption of its sugar, blunting those hunger-promoting spikes of blood glucose that sweets typically generate. And for some healthy icing on the cake, dark chocolate may even trick your body into burning more fat. The "active ingredients" for health and flavor in dark chocolate are a class of super-potent antioxidants called flavanols. Flavanols have been shown to enhance the action of insulin and boost metabolism while working all sorts of magic on the precious cells that line our blood vessels to keep blood flowing smoothly. So come over to the dark side and enjoy!

> "For best results, choose the highest cacao content your palate will accept (strive for at least 60%) and limit your indulgence to ⅓ to one ounce."

The Facts On...
COCOA

Cocoa powder is exploding with super-potent antioxidants called flavanols. Flavanols work all sorts of magic on blood vessels, keeping them open and functioning well. According to a recent clinical trial, enjoying a daily cup of hot cocoa made with skim milk can boost HDL (good cholesterol) and decrease proteins that trigger the development of artery plaque in as little as one month. Be sure to use 100% cocoa powder and stay away from the instant varieties.

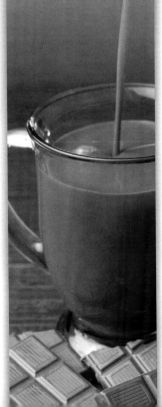

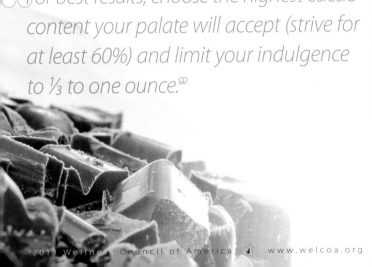

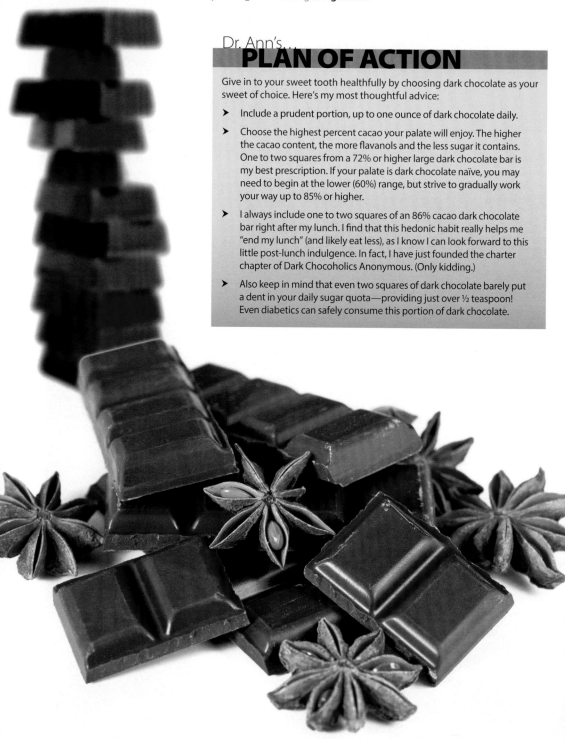

Dr. Ann's...
PLAN OF ACTION

Give in to your sweet tooth healthfully by choosing dark chocolate as your sweet of choice. Here's my most thoughtful advice:

➤ Include a prudent portion, up to one ounce of dark chocolate daily.

➤ Choose the highest percent cacao your palate will enjoy. The higher the cacao content, the more flavanols and the less sugar it contains. One to two squares from a 72% or higher large dark chocolate bar is my best prescription. If your palate is dark chocolate naïve, you may need to begin at the lower (60%) range, but strive to gradually work your way up to 85% or higher.

➤ I always include one to two squares of an 86% cacao dark chocolate bar right after my lunch. I find that this hedonic habit really helps me "end my lunch" (and likely eat less), as I know I can look forward to this little post-lunch indulgence. In fact, I have just founded the charter chapter of Dark Chocoholics Anonymous. (Only kidding.)

➤ Also keep in mind that even two squares of dark chocolate barely put a dent in your daily sugar quota—providing just over ½ teaspoon! Even diabetics can safely consume this portion of dark chocolate.

RESEARCH CORNER

Dark Chocolate Put To The Test

Scientists from the University of Copenhagen sought to compare the effects of milk chocolate vs. dark chocolate on feelings of fullness and subsequent food intake. In the study, 16 healthy males reported to the lab for two separate chocolate-eating sessions. They were fed 100 grams of dark chocolate or milk chocolate and monitored in the lab for the next five hours. During the course of that time, their feelings of fullness, hunger, and specific food cravings were noted.

Halfway through the five-hour period, the study participants were given pizza and instructed to eat until they felt comfortably satisfied. Study participants consumed 15% less calories of pizza after the dark chocolate than they did after the milk chocolate. They also reported less of a desire for sweet, salty, or fatty foods after the dark chocolate.

12 Reasons To Eat Dark Chocolate

I recently reviewed all of the studies I had in my files related to dark chocolate. I am ecstatic to report the following scientific accolades for this indulgence:

1. Enhances blood flow, including blood flow to the heart and brain

2. Lowers blood pressure

3. Improves the function and health of blood vessels

4. Lowers triglycerides

5. Raises HDL (good) cholesterol levels

6. Lowers LDL (bad) cholesterol levels

7. Reduces inflammation

8. Improves the action of the hormone insulin (which means better blood sugar metabolism)

9. Enhances cognitive function

10. Lowers the risk of heart disease and strokes

11. Improves longevity

12. Lifts mood and boosts energy

Tips For... HEALTHIER BAKING

My youngest daughter, Lucie, is aspiring to be the world's best "healthy" chef. She is only in ninth grade and well on her way. She loves to bake and wanted me to share these tips for healthier baking:

➤ Substitute canola oil for shortening, stick margarine, or butter. Canola oil/butter blends are also acceptable.

➤ Use ground flax seeds, ground nuts, or all natural nut butters in place of bad fats (butter, stick margarine, shortening).

➤ Replace butter with yogurt.

➤ Substitute whole wheat flour or white whole wheat flour ("Ultra-grain" King Arthur Brand®) for white flour.

➤ Use buttermilk (1% or nonfat) instead of milk or sour cream.

➤ Substitute plain Greek-style yogurt for sour cream.

➤ Substitute dark or semisweet chocolate for milk chocolate.

➤ Substitute pureed dates, honey, maple syrup, or molasses for sugar.

➤ To reduce the fat or butter in your recipes without compromising flavor, add nuts, spices (i.e. cinnamon), instant espresso powder, coffee, cocoa powder, dried fruit, extracts (i.e. vanilla), liqueurs (i.e. amaretto), citrus zests or juice, 100% fruit butters, or nut oils.

➤ To moisten and add nutritional value to baked goods, mix in 100% canned pumpkin or sweet potato puree, grated raw veggies (i.e. carrots), or smashed bananas.

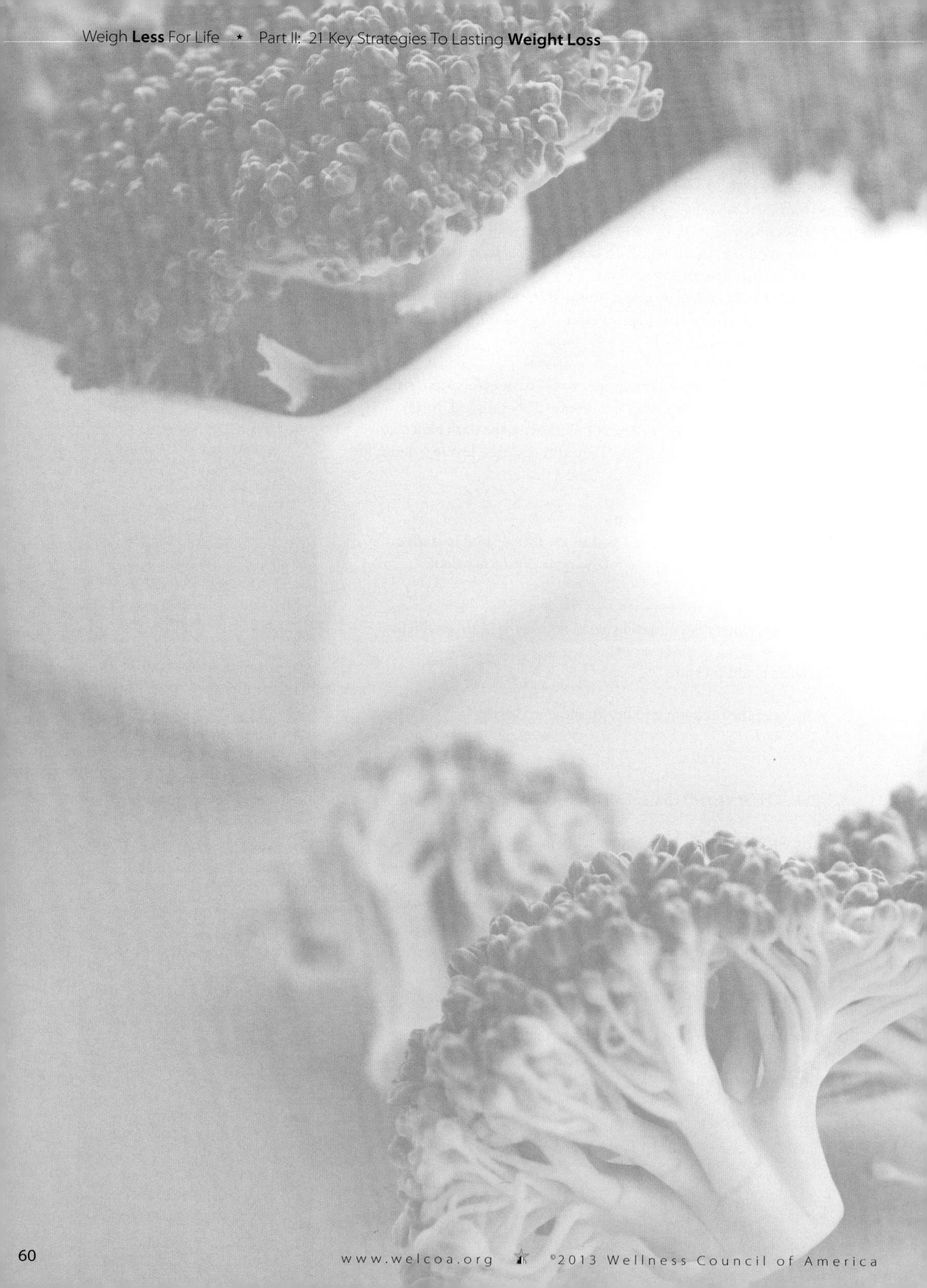

Keep Meals & Snacks
Flavor-Simple

Keep Meals & Snacks
Flavor-Simple

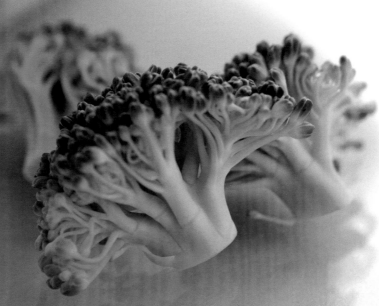

Most all of us could benefit from simplifying our lives, and I highly recommend doing the same with your food flavors. The reason is elemental—the greater the variety of flavors within a food or a meal, the more we want to eat.

This reality is due to something called sensory-specific satiety. Housed within our brain's appetite control center of the hypothalamus are areas that respond specifically to distinct flavors or tastes in foods, like sweet, salty, sour, and savory. This means that sweet tastes will stimulate one area, savory another, and so on.

When you eat, the flavor or flavors within that food will stimulate and awaken the corresponding flavor-specific area or areas within the hypothalamus. Once awakened, each taste-specific area releases the hunger-promoting hormone neuropeptide Y (NPY).

When it comes to hunger, NPY can be an enemy to any diet. This hormone is a particularly powerful appetite stimulator and prompts you to really want food. Turning on multiple areas of the appetite center simultaneously by eating various flavors at once means that the brain will release even more NPY. This leads to more intense appetite stimulation and food-seeking behavior, and ultimately increases the time it takes to feel full.

The food industry, which depends on food consumption for its livelihood, is well aware of this phenomenon and exploits it relentlessly. Almost every processed, bagged, wrapped, or boxed food on the grocery shelf is a virtual cornucopia of appetite-inciting flavors. With sweet, salty, savory, and sour, along with a spectacular array of newfangled artificial flavors commingling in endless combinations layer upon layer, it's no wonder that we are hungrier than ever—and consuming more than ever!

Research CORNER

The Findings On Flavor

In a series of two experiments, study subjects were offered either a variety of foods (multiple flavors) in succession within a given meal or the same food (one flavor) in succession for a meal. In both sessions, they were instructed to eat until they felt full. Food intakes were recorded and compared after all the test meals.

In the first meal, study subjects were either given sandwiches for lunch with four different-flavored fillings, or sandwiches with just one simple filling. When provided with the different fillings, the subjects ate 33% more than those who were offered just one filling.

In the second experiment, study subjects were offered either three flavors of yogurt or a single flavor. Here again, they ate significantly more when given the variety of flavored yogurts.

Dr. Ann's... PLAN OF ACTION

How do you break free from the food industry's endless flavor factory to eat healthier meals? The secret is to "simplify" by eating mostly whole, real, nature-made foods.

➤ Choose foods with as simple a flavor profile as possible.

➤ Avoid flavor-turbocharged, factory-made, processed foods. The longer a processed food's ingredients list, the more permissive it will be.

➤ Whole, fresh, unprocessed foods provided by nature will always be your very best choice. Fruits, veggies, beans, lean proteins, nuts, dairy, and whole grains rule.

➤ As a simple exercise to keep you on track, before you eat anything, ask yourself if your great-grandfather could have eaten it. If yes, it will likely be a good choice.

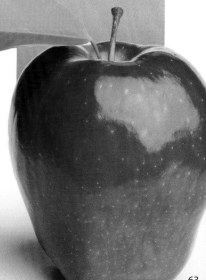

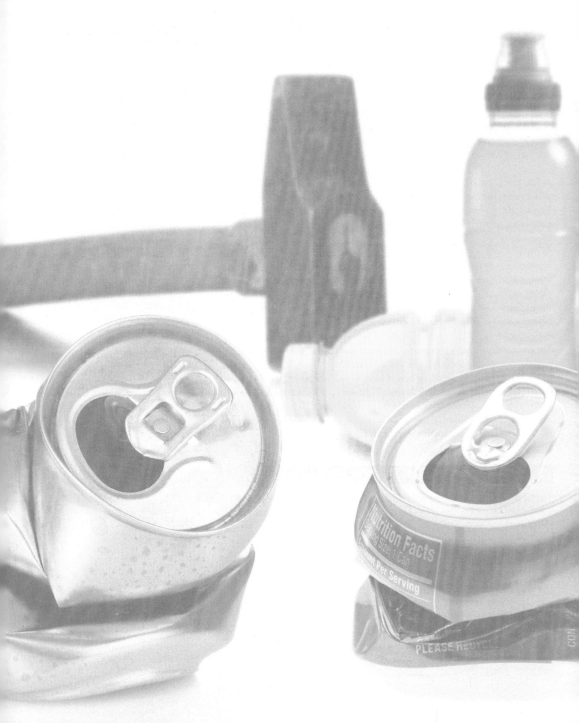

Dump All
Sugary Beverages

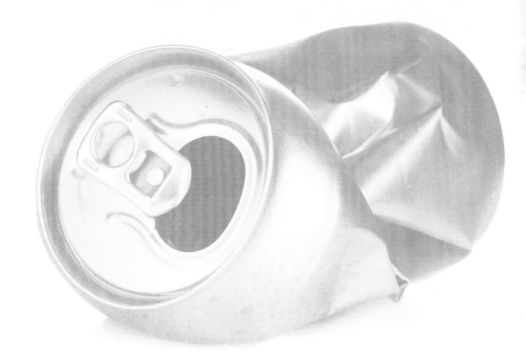

Dump All
Sugary Beverages

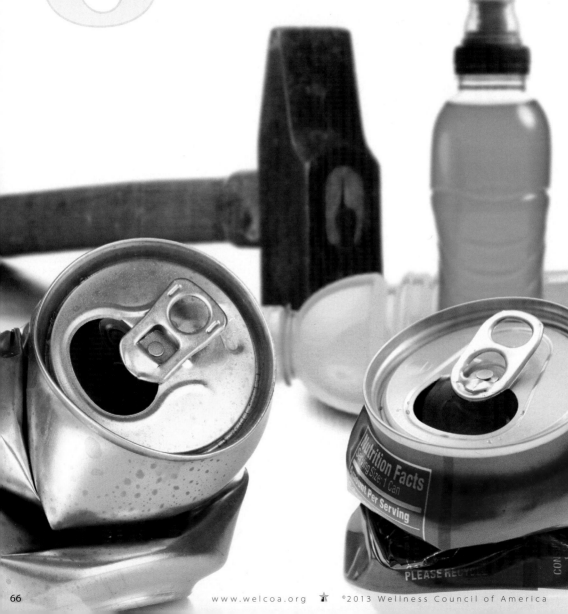

OF ALL THE THINGS YOU COULD DO TO CONSUME FEWER CALORIES, THE SIMPLE STEP OF DUMPING ANY SWEET DRINKS MIGHT OFFER THE SINGLE GREATEST RETURN FOR YOUR EFFORTS. Over the past several years, liquid calories, especially sugary beverages like soda and fruit drinks, have emerged as the most belly-boosting of all forms of calories. Unfortunately, sweetened beverages are now the number one source of calories in the toxic U.S. diet, and they have been consistently linked to weight gain, obesity, type 2 diabetes, and metabolic syndrome.

There are many different ways that sugary beverages can drown your diet. Because they lack physical bulk, liquids do not suppress appetite to the same degree as their solid-food counterparts. They simply do not "fill" the stomach and elicit the cascade of hunger-suppressing signals that real foods do.

When you consider the far-leaner times of our predecessors, the hunter-gatherers, it is perfectly understandable that "drinking" would not suppress appetite. For these ancient ancestors, zero-calorie water was the only beverage available. If taking in water decreased appetite, it would have diminished chances for survival by reducing the drive to seek food and thus acquire essential calories and nutrients. Scientists speculate that this likely explains why separate and distinct areas of the brain mediate hunger and thirst.

Whether you are partial to soda, fruit drinks, or decadent coffee drinks, remember that when you quench your thirst with one of these ubiquitous beverages, you are consuming a hefty dose of concentrated sugar—sugar that zips straight to your bloodstream as a flash flood of glucose and fructose. The "twin peaks" of glucose and fructose are notorious for appetite stimulation and for disrupting metabolism. Finally, sipping rather than chewing provides less opportunity for orosensory satiety, or in plain English, satisfying the "cravings of your mouth," and makes it considerably easier to take in excess calories quickly and effortlessly.

The result? A perfect storm of easy calories that do absolutely nothing to satisfy your hunger.

Thankfully, there is some good news in all of this. Reducing your intake of sweetened beverages appears to have a larger impact on weight reduction than reducing the equivalent amount of solid-food calories. Studies have also shown that eliminating liquid calories does not seem to make us hungrier, as is the case with cutting out solid-food calories.

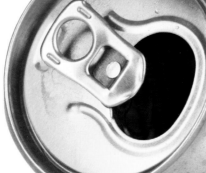

Coconut Water: Nature's Sports Drink

Thanks to a new scientific analysis, it appears that coconut water can rightly claim its reputation as Mother Nature's sports drink. Coconut water is the clear liquid harvested from young green coconuts and is now available at many grocery outlets and health food stores.

Researchers analyzed all the components in coconut water relative to those in comparable amounts of Gatorade® and PowerAde® and found that coconut water provides five times more potassium, equivalent amounts of magnesium and carbohydrates, and about one-third less sodium.

Additionally, coconut water contained high levels of beneficial antioxidants (not found in the other sports drinks) and fewer calories, and sugar. The researchers did note that those engaged in prolonged, strenuous exercise accompanied by heavy sweating may need additional sodium to replace their losses.

Coconut water is always my sports beverage of choice, and if I think I need more sodium—I add a pinch of salt.

Dr. Ann's...
PLAN OF ACTION

Here are my instructions for losing the liquids.

➤ Choose zero-calorie, 100% healthy water as your beverage of choice.

➤ If you enjoy them, include 100% vegetable or tomato juice, unsweetened coffee or tea freely, 1% or skim milk, or plain soy milk in moderation.

➤ Strictly avoid all sweet beverages including: soda, fruit drinks, fruit juice, sweet tea, energy drinks, and any others sweet beverages that venture on the scene.

➤ Don't forget about dessert and specialty coffee drinks. A 16-ounce frappuccino provides an eye-popping 500+ calories. Ditto for most store-bought smoothies.

➤ While diet beverages provide little to no calories, they are not a healthy substitute and may come along with their own risks for weight gain. At a minimum, sugar substitutes keep our highly permissive taste buds for sweetness on overdrive.

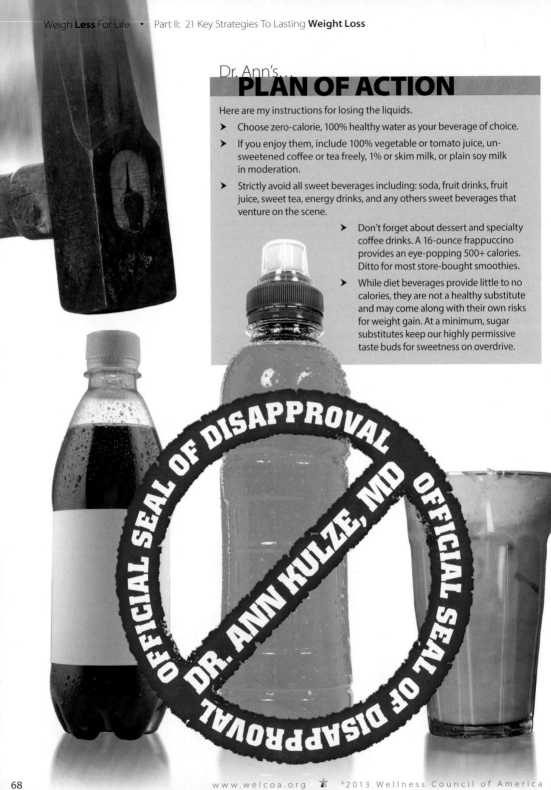

OFFICIAL SEAL OF DISAPPROVAL DR. ANN KULZE, MD OFFICIAL SEAL OF DISAPPROVAL

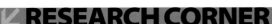

RESEARCH CORNER

The Impact Of Liquid Calories

The dangers of sugary beverages are well documented in research. Here are two to wet your appetite.

In a landmark report from the esteemed Harvard Nurse's Health Study, investigators followed the drinking habits of over 51,000 women from 1991 to 1995. In this investigation, drinking sugary beverages was strongly associated with taking in excess calories and weight gain.

Over a four-year period, study subjects who increased their intake of sugary beverages from less than one a week to one or more a day increased their calories by 358 per day. This same group gained over 10 pounds over the four-year study period.

The researchers concluded that the association between weight gain and sugary beverages was likely due to the large amount of quickly absorbable sugars the beverages provide, along with their propensity to readily push people into positive caloric balance.

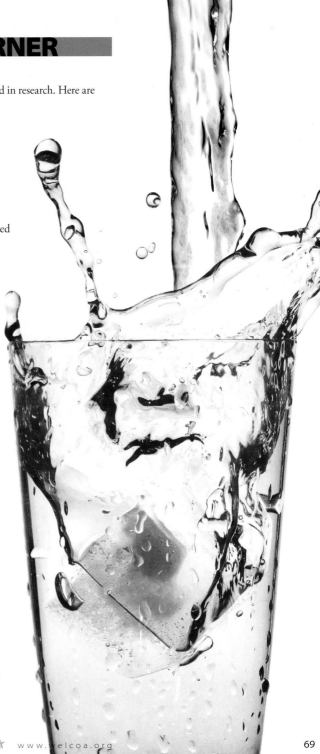

A recent review of 88 published studies showed a solid and consistent link between soda consumption and obesity, diabetes, and poor nutrition. One of the most shocking findings was a study of more than 91,000 women that found those who drank one or more sodas per day (keep in mind, this is less than the U.S. national average) were two times more likely to develop diabetes vs. those who drank less than one per month. Given that sugar-sweetened beverages (primarily soda) currently make up the single greatest source of calories for Americans—it's no wonder that type 2 diabetes is currently the runaway train. Curiously, the scientist who reviewed these 88 studies reported a "remarkable difference" in study results depending upon whether the study was industry or non-industry sponsored. I'll play it safe and stick to my water!

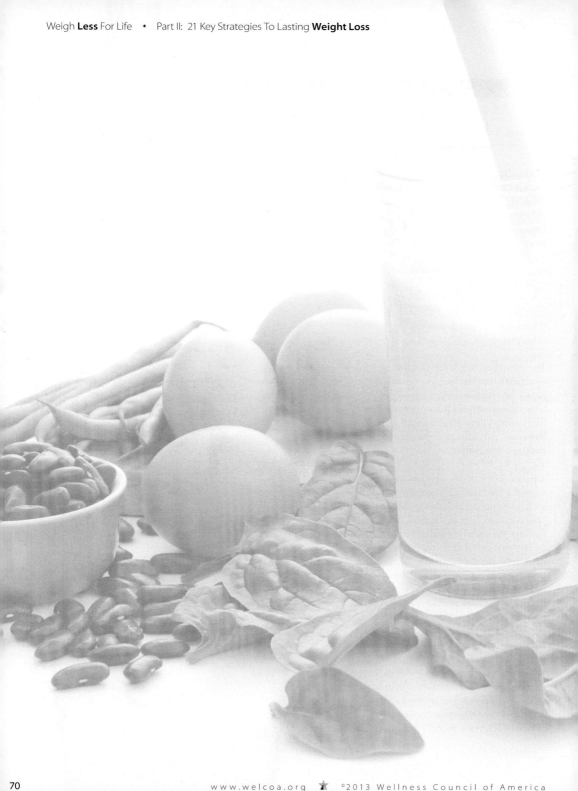

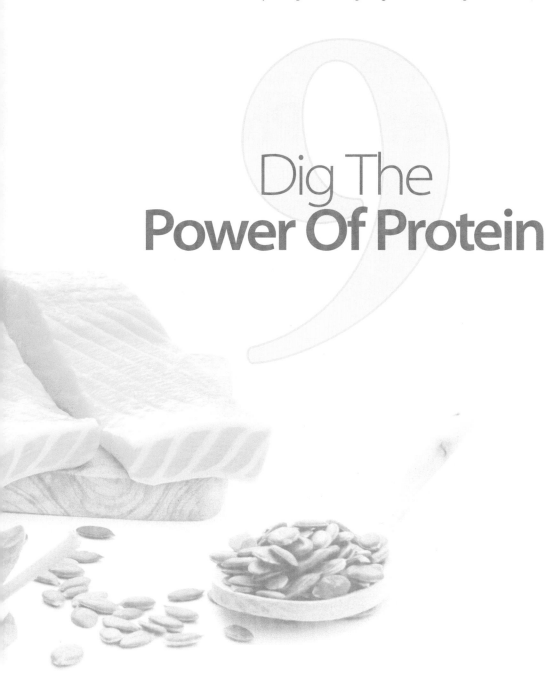

Dig The
Power Of Protein

Dig The
Power Of Protein

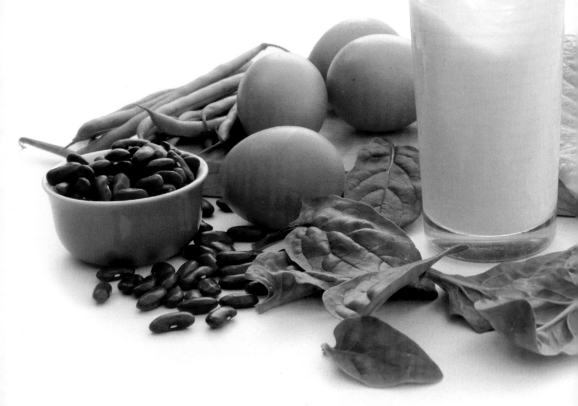

O F THE THREE BASIC BUILDING BLOCKS OF NUTRITION—PROTEIN, CARBOHYDRATES, AND FAT—NOTHING PROVIDES LONGER-LASTING AND MORE EFFECTIVE APPETITE CONTROL THAN PROTEIN. In fact, I like to call protein nature's diet pill!

While the uniquely sating power of protein has not been conclusively elucidated, there are a number of potential mechanisms at play. When proteins are digested, they produce a more prolonged and steady level of glucose in the bloodstream. This can keep the appetite center in your glucose-loving brain stuck in the "off" position longer than it would be if you were to eat a carbohydrate or fat-laden meal. Foods that are rich in protein also slow down the overall digestive process by delaying gastric emptying. This means that foods will stay in your stomach longer, enhancing the feeling of fullness and satiety. Protein has also been shown to drive down the levels of ghrelin more effectively than the equivalent calories from carbs and fats. Ghrelin is a hormone produced in the cells that line the stomach and functions as the body's most powerful appetite-stimulating hormone. It bangs on the brain's dinner bell and drives food-seeking behavior. There is even laboratory evidence that the building blocks of protein, called amino acids, directly stimulate specialized brain cells that prompt us to stay alert and burn more calories. This may explain why people report feeling more energized after protein-rich vs. carb-rich meals.

If you are trying to lose weight, getting optimal protein can also help preserve your muscle mass. This is very important because dieting can lead to loss of muscle, which slows metabolism and reduces functionality.

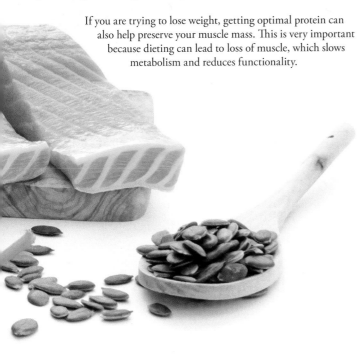

Stay Strong!

Maintaining muscle mass is fundamental to a healthy metabolism and essential for optimal functionality. The International Osteoporosis Foundation recently sought to review past worldwide studies to identify the most effective nutritional avenues for preventing loss of muscle mass, known as sarcopenia. The following key strategies were identified:

1. **Focus on optimal protein intake:** As we age, it takes higher doses of protein to stimulate muscle protein synthesis. Unfortunately, most people eat less, not more protein as they age. The ideal intake of daily protein based on this evaluation was 1 to 1.2 grams/kilogram of body weight a day. For clearer perspective—that is about ½ your body weight in pounds. In other words, if you weigh 150 pounds you would need 75 grams of protein a day. Based on my experience, I would estimate that less than 10% of the elderly are getting optimal intakes of protein for maintaining or building muscle. Those with kidney disease need to consult with their healthcare provider about optimal protein requirements.

(Continued on page 74.)

Stay Strong!

(Continued from page 73.)

2. Ensure you maintain an adequate vitamin D intake: Vitamin D plays a pivotal role in preservation of muscle mass and muscle function. To ensure adequate intakes, get regular, safe sun exposure, consume vitamin D rich foods regularly (fortified dairy products, eggs, and oily fish), and take a daily vitamin D supplement. I recommend 2000 IU's of vitamin D3 a day for adults or as directed by your healthcare provider based on your blood level measurements.

3. Aim for an alkaline-based diet as opposed to an acid-based diet: Meats, sweets, and processed grains and carbohydrates give rise to acidic metabolic by-products. Consuming fruits and veggies provides an alkalizing effect in the body. For best results, consume an abundance of fruits and veggies while restricting meats, sweets, and processed foods.

4. Consider B vitamin supplements. There is growing evidence that vitamin B12 and folic acid are also important for maintaining muscle mass and strength. If you are age 50 or older, get your blood levels periodically checked to be sure you do not need supplements.

Please also note that resistance exercise (yoga, bands, Pilates, free weights, and weight machines) is essential for maintaining muscle mass with aging and the most powerful of all muscle-preserving strategies! Strive for 15-20 minutes (that is about a minute a muscle) twice a week.

Dr. Ann's...
PLAN OF ACTION

To give hunger the boot and help you preserve or build lean body mass, the secret is to get enough protein at each of your three meals. Here are some strategies that will help you in that effort.

➤ Include a nice dose of protein at each meal. Strive for at least 15 grams, but 25 to 30 grams (especially for men) is likely best. For further guidance, note that lean animal proteins (fish, poultry, red meat) generally provide about 21 grams per 3 ounces (about the size of a deck of cards); a cup of milk 8 grams; a cup of beans about 17 grams; an individual container of low-fat Greek yogurt 15 grams; a large egg 7 grams; ½ cup tofu 9 grams; and 2 tbsp peanut butter 8 grams. The right dose of protein should give you at least 2 to 2½ hours of satiety.

➤ If you are hungry less than two hours after a meal, chances are you need to step up the protein a bit. Or perhaps you ate too many Great White Hazards!

➤ The best protein choices for your health and your waistline include fish, shellfish, skinless poultry, nuts, peanut or other nut butters, seeds, whole soy foods, low-fat or skim dairy products, omega-3 eggs, and beans/legumes. Of course you can include multiple protein sources at mealtime as desired to help you reach your quota.

➤ Getting adequate protein at breakfast appears to be especially valuable for appetite control—even for later in the day. So be particularly attentive to protein at breakfast. (See page 79.)

RESEARCH CORNER

Protein Put To The Test

To specifically test the notion that protein is superior for appetite control, researchers at the University of Washington School of Medicine placed 19 study subjects sequentially on different diets, each varying in protein content.

In the first phase, the study subjects were placed on a two-week weight-maintenance diet. On that diet, 15% of calories came from protein, 35% came from fat, and 50% came from carbohydrates.

In phase 2, they were transitioned to a two-week diet consisting of the same number of calories, but with more protein and less fat (30% from protein, 20% from fat, and 50% from carbohydrates). Then the study subjects spent the final 12-week phase eating whatever they wanted, while maintaining the same percentages of calories from foods (again, 30% from protein, 20% from fat, and 50% from carbs).

The results? Study subjects reported a markedly decreased appetite while on the higher protein diet of phase 2 vs. the lower protein phase 1. Additionally, during

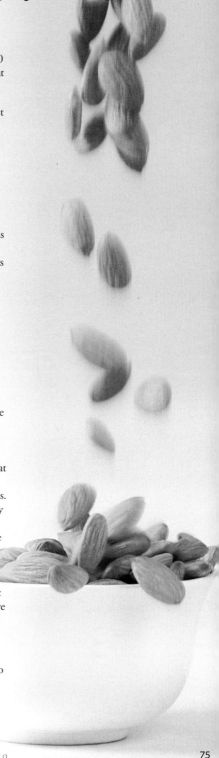

phase 3, despite the fact that they could eat whatever they wanted, they ate 450 less calories daily and lost 11 pounds on average. The investigators concluded that "calorie for calorie" protein provides a greater sense of satiety than carbs or fat.

In a recent clinical trial, scientists placed study subjects on three different test diets each with varying levels of protein—either 10%, 15% or 25 % protein. The study subjects who were fed the 10% protein diet ate 12% more calories over the 4-day study period (mostly from increased snacking) vs. when they were fed the 15% protein diet. There was no difference however in calorie intake on the 15% protein diet vs. the 25% protein diet. The researchers concluded that humans have a particularly strong appetite for protein and when protein needs are not met—hunger and excess eating can ensue.

For someone on a 2,000 calorie a day diet—15% protein translates to 75 grams of protein a day or about 25 grams per meal. For optimal weight control, be sure to have your protein and eat it too. The amount of protein in the diet plays an influential role in how many total calories are consumed over the day.

The Best Way To Eat For Weight Loss

In a landmark report that comprised the "world's largest diet study"— researchers concluded that the most effective dietary regimen for preventing and treating obesity is one that is relatively high in lean protein (25% of calories) and low in its glycemic response. Glycemic response refers to how high and how fast the carbs you eat raise your blood sugar. The researchers placed 773 adults and their children (a total of 827 kids) on one of five types of eating plans. The group on the high protein/low glycemic regime had the most success. One of the most remarkable findings was that the children in the families assigned to this type of eating experienced a spontaneous drop in the prevalence of overweight from 46% to 39%. This occurred with no dieting, no calorie counting, and no limits on the amounts of foods consumed. The restrictions were simply on the types or qualitative aspects of the foods served at home. The proteins consumed in these high protein/low glycemic households were lean meats, poultry, seafood, low-fat dairy products, eggs, beans, and nuts. The carbohydrates were of a low to moderate glycemic index and included: any vegetables except potatoes and corn; physically intact or coarse whole grains like oatmeal, brown rice, and whole grain bread with lots of kernels; temperate fruits like berries, apples, and pears with limits on tropical fruits like bananas, pineapple and mango. High glycemic carbohydrates, namely white rice, white potatoes, white flour products and sugary foods/sweets were restricted. Given what we now know about how protein and carbs with varying glycemic response impact appetite, this is not at all surprising, but it is wonderful to have such powerful science to back it up.

Appetite control is the Holy Grail for achieving and maintaining a healthy body weight. The best way to control your appetite is to eat lean protein at your meals, along with an abundance of low glycemic carbs and minimal to no Great White Hazards (white flour products, white rice, white potatoes, sugar/sweets).

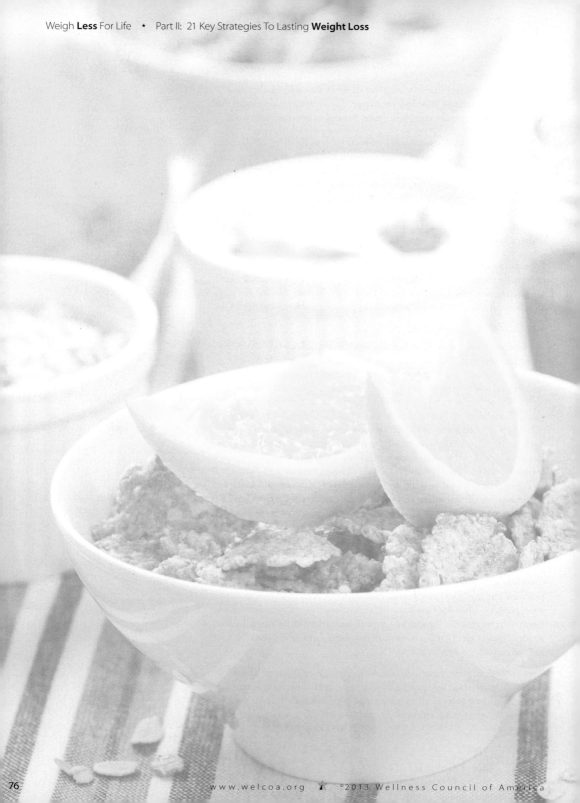

Never Skip **Breakfast!**

Never Skip
Breakfast!

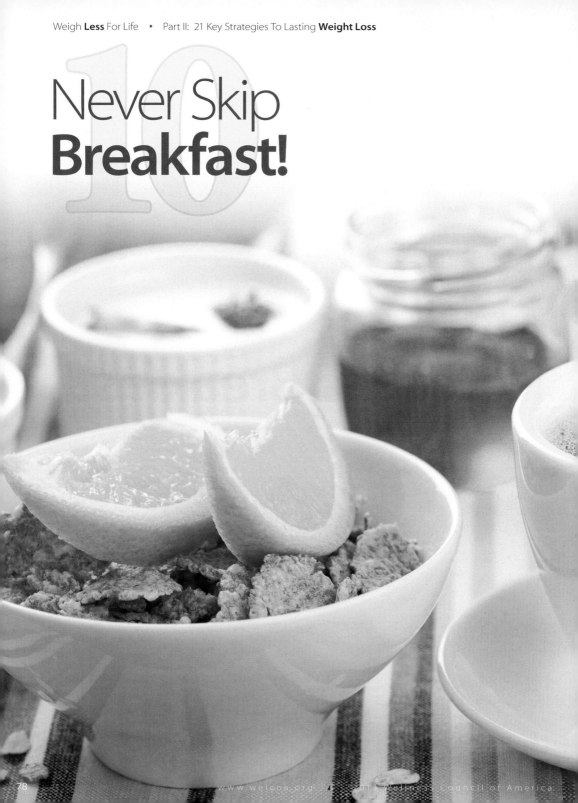

For what seem like ages now, we have all heard that breakfast is the most important ingredient in the recipe for an energized, productive day. But that's not all that breakfast has going for it. According to a large body of science, eating breakfast regularly aids in weight loss and weight control. Conversely, scientists consistently observe that people who skip this meal are significantly more likely to become overweight and suffer from metabolic issues.

There are several logical reasons why eating breakfast is good for the waistline, including kick-starting metabolism and boosting energy expenditure. But reason number one is simple: Breakfast helps us eat less throughout the remainder of the day.

Skipping breakfast after the "fasting period" of nightly sleep naturally ramps up appetite, compelling us toward dietary indiscretions and even binging. Studies show regular breakfast skippers (currently about 20% of the population) snack more, crave and eat more high-calorie, high-risk foods like chips, sodas, and sweets (especially at night), and get less nutrients over the day than those who take advantage of a morning feeding. In the semi-starved state of no breakfast, the brain is especially primed for appetite activation. Even the slightest environmental provocation like a TV commercial with risky foods will compel you to seek them out—so be forewarned! What's more, recent research has shown that after skipping a meal, the foods we naturally go for first at the next meal are starchy carbs, and the foods we begin a meal with are the ones we eat the most of. This can add insult to injury.

Lastly, in terms of appetite and eating behavior, self-control seems to be greatest during the early parts of the day. If you do eat breakfast, this makes it easier to fill up in the morning on healthy, prudent, good-for-appetite-control foods like lean protein, fiber-rich produce, and whole grains. Studies show that a nice dose of protein at breakfast can be especially valuable for appetite control over the remainder of the day. So be particularly diligent in including some healthy protein with your breakfast. And of course, just say NO! to any Great White Hazard appetite stimulants like muffins, pastries, waffles, and white flour bagels.

Research CORNER

Eat Your Breakfast And Don't Forget Your Protein

To evaluate the impact of breakfast on appetite, researchers had a group of teens skip breakfast daily for three weeks or eat a normal or higher protein breakfast daily for three weeks. Throughout the study, subjects answered questionnaires about their feelings of hunger and satiety. In addition, each subject had a brain scan prior to lunch to identify levels of activation in appetite-driving areas of the brain. Relative to breakfast skippers, those consuming both the regular and higher protein breakfast reported less hunger throughout the morning. Consistent with their subjective responses, the brain scans of the breakfast eaters revealed reduced activation in brain areas involved in food motivation. As anticipated, the higher protein breakfast eaters had the greatest reduction in appetite and brain activation throughout the study.

Dr. Ann's... PLAN OF ACTION

Simply committing to eat breakfast every day is the important first step. Here are some additional tips to get your morning and your appetite off on the right foot.

➤ For optimal results, be sure that your breakfast includes some protein and fiber-rich carbohydrates.

➤ Logical breakfast proteins include the following, alone or in any combination that works for you: plain soy milk, skim or 1% milk, peanut butter, almond butter, smoked or canned salmon, low-fat or non-fat Greek-style yogurt, cottage cheese, omega-3 eggs, part-skim or 2% milk cheeses, high-protein cereals, protein powder (great in smoothies), and nuts or seeds. The right dose of breakfast protein should keep your hunger under wraps for two to three full hours. Step it up as needed.

➤ Good sources of fiber-rich breakfast carbohydrates include: high-fiber cereals (five grams or more per serving), oatmeal (preferably steel-cut), fresh or frozen fruits, and vegetables (think a veggie omelet, or salsa on top of eggs).

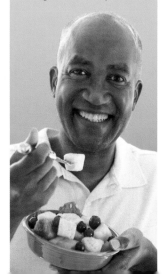

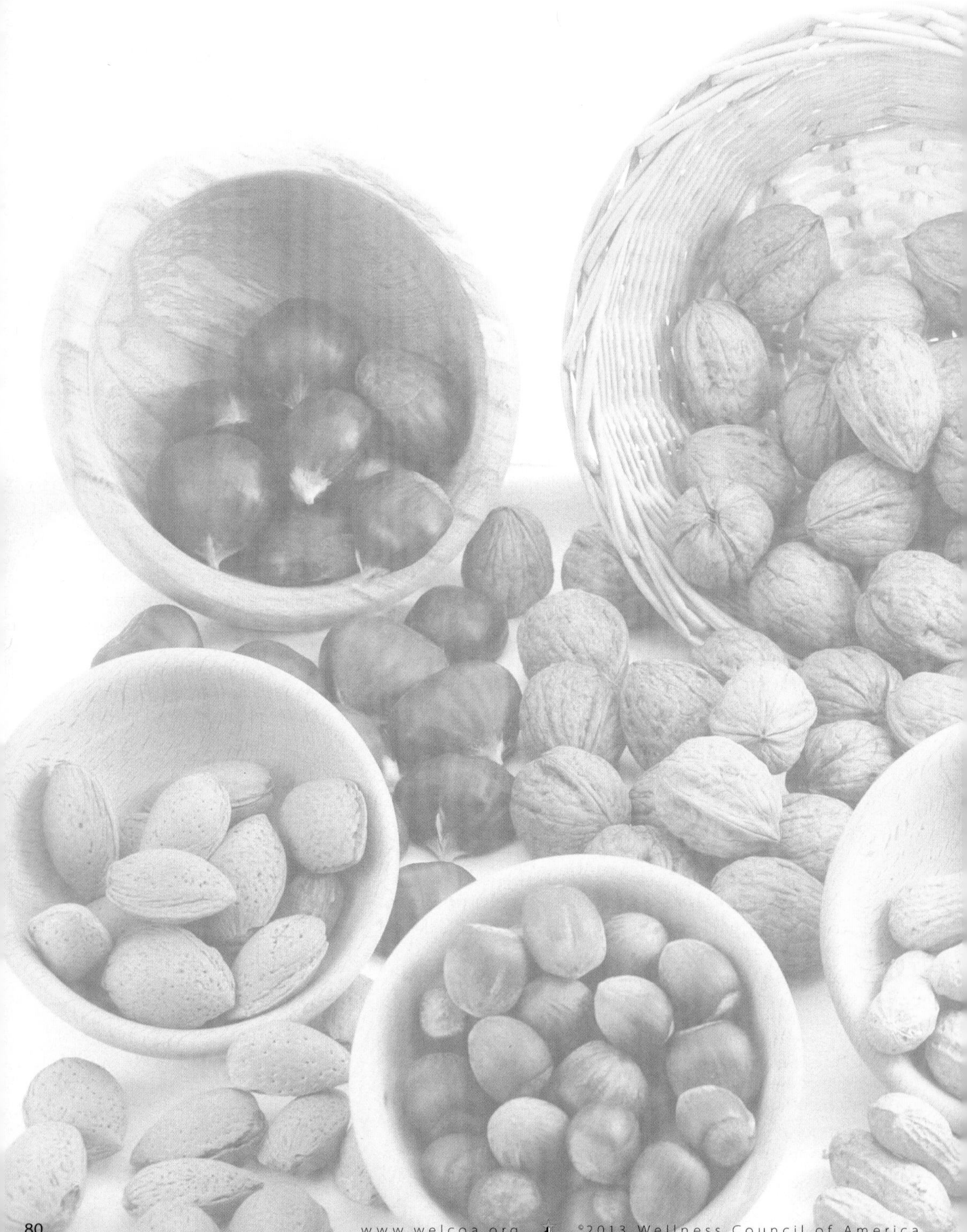

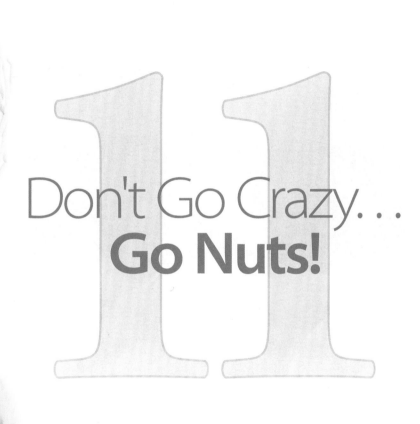

Don't Go Crazy...
Go Nuts!

Don't Go Crazy. . .
Go Nuts!

11

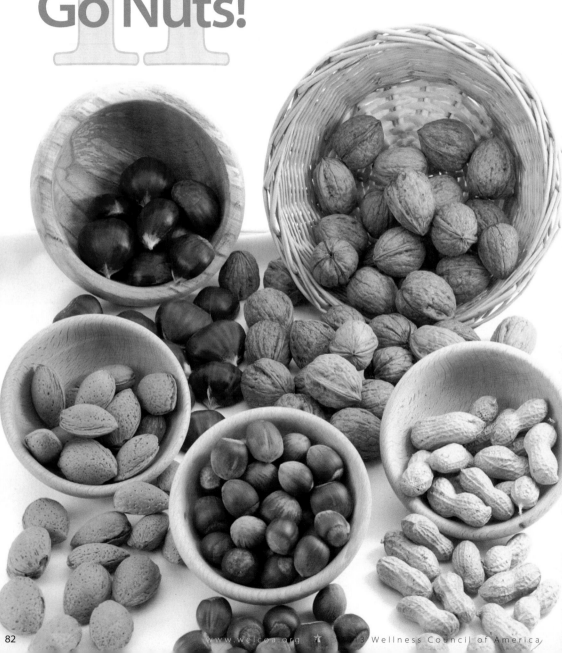

WHEN IT COMES TO THE DUAL QUALITIES OF HEALTH PROTECTION AND APPETITE CONTROL, NUTS SCORE A PERFECT 10. These delectable morsels are exploding with nutritional firepower. They provide stellar cardiovascular protection, guard against type 2 diabetes and macular degeneration, and are a standout food for longevity and fighting inflammation.

Nuts also provide a truly delicious way to help you eat less. Studies consistently show that people who include nuts regularly in their diets are healthier and leaner, than those who don't.

Do nuts contain some special fat-burning ingredient? Likely not, but they do offer that terrific trio of protein, fiber, and fat that provides quick appetite suppression (from the fat), along with a sustained feeling of fullness (from the protein and fiber).

Nuts are also high in the heart-healthy monounsaturated fat, oleic acid. As fats go, oleic acid has the unique ability to directly stimulate the release of a special "feel-full" hormone, OEA, from the small intestine. OEA makes its way directly into the brain and turns on circuits that make you feel fuller for longer. Additionally, relative to other fats, oleic acid tends to give rise to a more exuberant release of appetite-quieting hormones from the GI tract.

Dr. Ann's...
PLAN OF ACTION

To shore up your health and your appetite control—eat nuts regularly.

➤ Include a moderate handful (about 1 ounce) of nuts in your diet each day. For perspective, an ounce of nuts is about 20 almonds or 12 walnut halves. If weight is not an issue, include them as you desire.

➤ Choose the nuts that you enjoy, but strive for variety as they all have unique nutritional attributes.

➤ Your options include Brazil nuts, hazel nuts, almonds, pecans, walnuts, pistachios, pine nuts, macadamias, cashews, and peanuts.

➤ Peanuts and almonds have the most protein and may be a particularly good choice for appetite control.

➤ Try nuts as a mid-afternoon snack. It's the perfect way to make nuts part of your daily eating regimen.

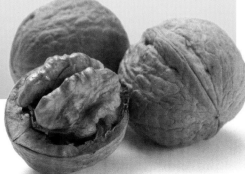

Research
CORNER

Nuts About Research

Delicious and nutritious nuts definitely pass muster in scientific circles. Honestly, the research behind nuts is simply glorious. Here are a couple of reports to crunch on.

To determine if eating nuts could reduce the risk of weight gain and obesity over the long term, Spanish researchers followed the diets of over 8,865 adults for a period of two years. Study subjects who reported consuming nuts two or more times per week gained significantly less weight over the two-year study than those who rarely or never ate nuts.

And just when I thought it could not get any better, scientists have uncovered yet another reason to go nuts for nuts. Past studies had indicated that nuts provide protection against metabolic syndrome (MetS) and weight gain, so scientists sought to investigate if eating nuts could lead to measurable improvements in the standard markers of metabolic health. For the study they placed 21 MetS patients on a nut-enriched diet (about an ounce or handful a day) and compared them to a control group of MetS patients who did not eat nuts. At the end of the study, the nut eaters experienced several measurable improvements in metabolic health. An intriguing and unexpected finding was that the nut eaters had an increase in their serotonin levels. Serotonin is the body's "feel happy" hormone and also plays a role in quieting appetite. In a nutshell—nuts are "real" good mood foods that are great for your waistline and your health!

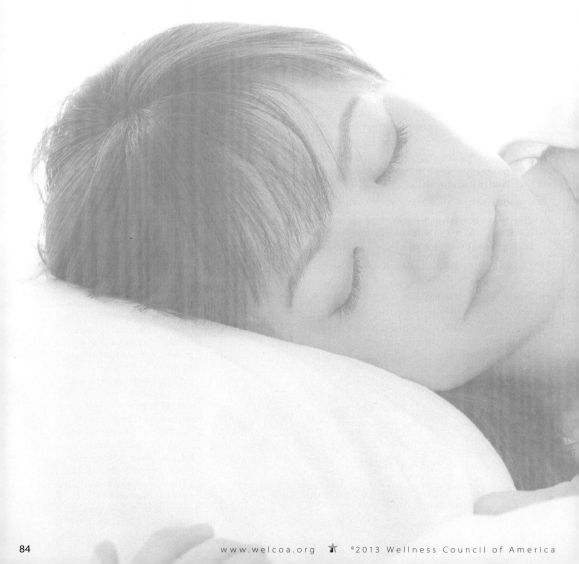

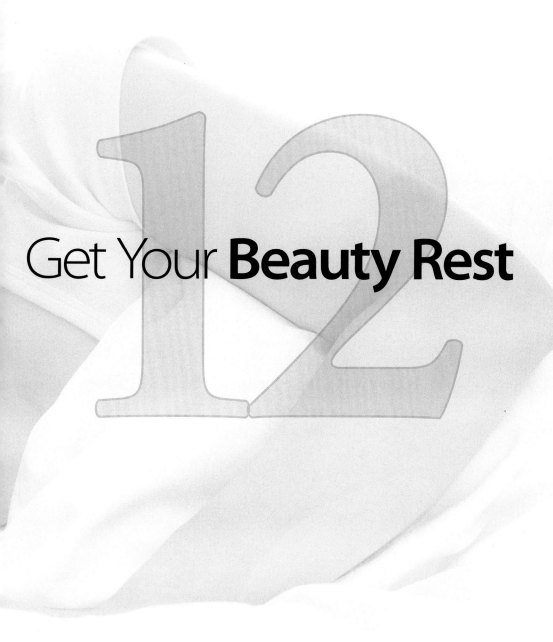

Get Your **Beauty Rest**

Get Your
Beauty Rest

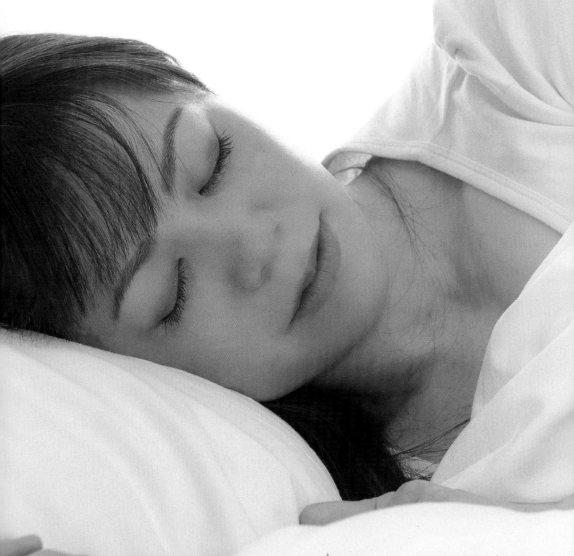

In SURVEY AFTER SURVEY, THE RESULTS ARE CLEAR—AND ALARMING: PEOPLE ARE SLEEPING LESS THAN EVER BEFORE. At the same time, our waistlines continue to grow larger and larger.

We now know these two facts are not merely coincidental. An ever-growing body of solid science is showing that sleep impacts body weight through a number of means, including appetite control. Recent research has uncovered that too little shut-eye elicits hormonal changes that boost hunger via a "double-whammy" mechanism. Let me explain.

After sleep deprivation, levels of the potent hunger-boosting hormone ghrelin increase, while levels of the hunger-quieting hormone leptin decrease. As would be expected given these hormonal changes, scientists also observe that poor sleep increases cravings for foods particularly apt to lead to weight gain, like donuts, cakes, and French fries. Unfortunately higher ghrelin levels have also been shown to reduce energy expenditure and promote fat retention. Sleep loss also impairs self-control (fundamental to eating less if you live in America), reduces motivation to exercise (as well as your energy level), and disrupts metabolism. In summation—inadequate sleep can make you fat and dramatically hinder your efforts to lose weight!

Dr. Ann's...
PLAN OF ACTION

Fortunately, there are some easy ways to prevent sleep deprivation from putting a damper on your diet. Here's what I suggest:

➤ Strive to get at least seven hours of restful sleep a night. Some people do even better with eight.

➤ Make the room you sleep in as dark, cool, and quiet as possible. Also keep it free of any electronics that can emit light or noise like a TV, tablet, phone, or computer.

➤ Avoid exercise or eating within two hours before bed, as these can stimulate you and prevent restful sleep.

➤ Try a soothing chamomile tea, meditating, or another relaxing practice that works for you to get your head and body ready for bed. Sex has been shown to encourage more restful sleep.

➤ Strive to maintain the same sleep and awaken times day to day.

➤ Avoid close exposure to the backlighting from a computer, tablet, or smart phone in the hour or two before bed. One recent study noted a significant decrease in the release of the sleep-inducing hormone melatonin from this artificial light.

➤ Get regular daily exercise. I am convinced that restful sleep is virtually impossible without a certain threshold level of daily physical activity (at least 30 minutes of moderate aerobic activity like brisk walking).

➤ Minimize the use of prescription sleep aids. They do not allow for restful, "normal" sleep and can predispose one to dependence.

Research
CORNER

How Sleep Affects Hunger

The impact of sleep on how we eat is very real. In fact, the chemical changes within the body tell the true story. Investigators measured the levels of the appetite-regulating hormones leptin and ghrelin in 12 men after a period of sleep deprivation and after a period of sufficient sleep. They also recorded the study subjects' hunger ratings after both periods. After two concurrent nights of just four hours of sleep, levels of the appetite-suppressive hormone leptin were 18% lower on average, while levels of the appetite-boosting hormone ghrelin were 28% higher compared to two nights of 10 hours of sleep. Similarly, the study subjects' hunger ratings increased by 24% after the sleep deprivation, and the foods they wanted the most were sweets, salty junk foods (chips), and starches (pastas and breads).

In a second study, one group of healthy adults got two consecutive nights of 10 hours of sleep, followed by five nights of restricted (four hours) sleep, and then four nights of normal (recovery) sleep. A second group got 10 concurrent nights of 10 hours of sleep. The sleep-deprived group gained an average of 2.9 pounds during the study period, while the other group did not experience any significant weight gain.

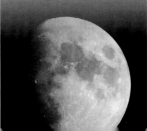

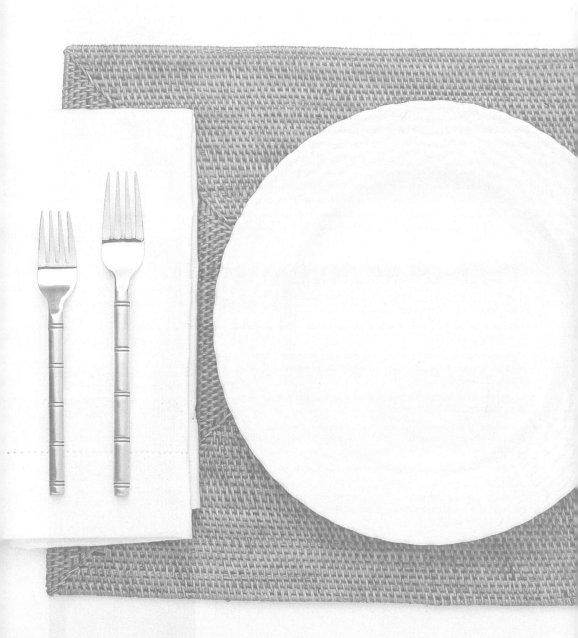

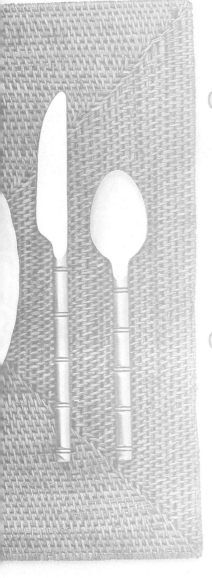

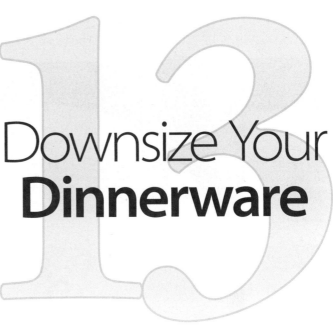

Downsize Your
Dinnerware

Downsize Your **Dinnerware**

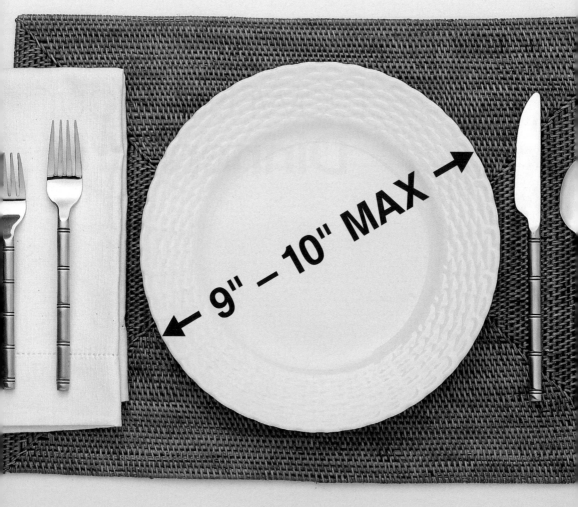

9" – 10" MAX

SOMETIMES, EATING LESS AND LOSING WEIGHT JUST COMES DOWN TO BASIC MATHEMATICS. And that's especially true at the dinner table. Here's the simple truth: The smaller our plates, bowls, and eating utensils, the less we serve ourselves and the less we eat.

Solid research has shown that smaller dinnerware can have a big impact. The size of a dish, along with your fork and spoon, is a powerful yet subversive cue when it comes to eating behavior. Simply stated, the larger our plates and serving pieces, the more we pile on (because we can), and the more we tend to eat. In essence, the practice of eating from smaller dishes builds in a reliable form of automatic portion control. After all, if you have less room, you're obviously going to give yourself less food.

But there's also a psychological game at work here, too. If you see a small bowl or plate that's full—as opposed to a large plate that's half empty—it naturally appears more appealing and provides a greater sense of satisfaction on the front end in contrast to one that appears sparse and puny. If your brain anticipates that a meal will fill you up, it automatically boosts the reality for true satiety.

History, in addition to science, seems to support this notion of smaller dinnerware equaling less food consumption. In the mid 1960s, the standard dinner plate was nine inches across. Now, the measurement is a whopping 12 inches! Surely it's no coincidence that our waistlines have expanded as well.

Dr. Ann's...
PLAN OF ACTION

To take advantage of the secrets of small, make the transition to eating off of smaller dishes and using smaller utensils. Here are some hints that can help.

➤ Retire your super-sized, modern dishes, and replace them with smaller versions.

➤ You can pick up vintage dinnerware and flatware from a local secondhand store or antique mall.

➤ Or, do what I do, and simply use a salad plate for your dinner plate, a dessert bowl in place of your regular bowl, and a teaspoon in place of a standard spoon.

Research
CORNER

We All Scream For Small Dishes!

To prove the validity of downsizing dinnerware to eat less, Cornell University researchers invited students and faculty from the department of nutrition to an "ice cream social." Invitees were randomly provided with a small or a large bowl and a small or a large serving spoon to dip their own ice cream.

The participants given the larger bowls ate over 30% more ice cream than those given the smaller bowls. In addition, those with larger spoons and a smaller bowl ate 15% more than those given smaller versions of both.

But the sprinkle on the ice cream was this: Those who used both the large bowl and the large spoon ate a gluttonous 57% more ice cream than those with the small spoon and bowl. The researchers concluded that the size of the dishes and serving utensils serves as a visual bias that can lead people to overeat.

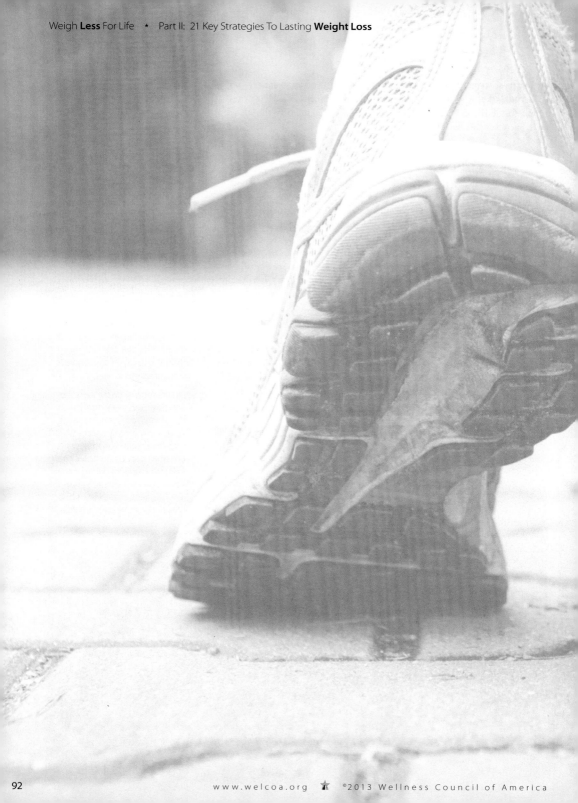

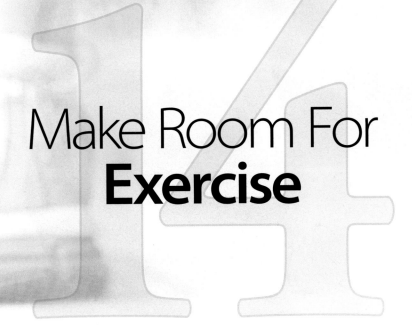

Make Room For
Exercise

Make Room For
Exercise

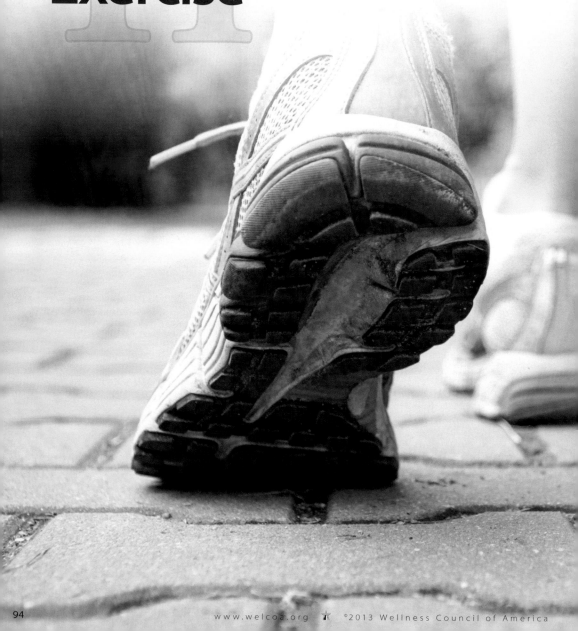

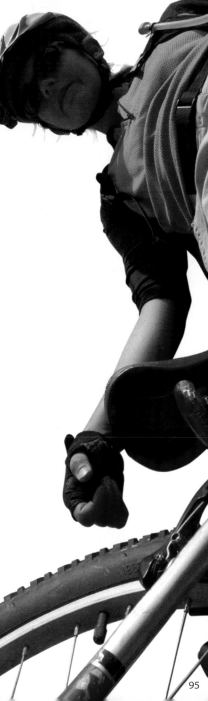

WHILE EXERCISE'S ABILITY TO BURN CALORIES AND JUMP-START METABOLISM IS COMMON KNOWLEDGE—DID YOU KNOW IT CAN QUIET YOUR APPETITE, TOO? Past studies have consistently shown that vigorous exercise, like running or spinning, provides a transient, but significant suppression of appetite. And scientists have now documented changes in appetite-control hormone levels during and after vigorous activity that nicely explain their observations. Perhaps even more exciting, especially for those who prefer moderate activity like brisk walking, even lighter forms of exercise seem to have a beneficial effect on appetite control at the level of the brain. It seems that moderate exercise can increase the sensitivity and responses of brain cells to the all-important appetite-quieting hormone leptin. Exercise has also been shown to diminish the brain's hunger-arousal response to visualizing images of appetizing, high-risk foods. Add in the undeniable fact that regular exercise, through its unbeatable stress-relieving effects, safeguards against emotional eating—and anyone can see that regular exercise is a sure-fire winner for helping us eat less!

Eight Reasons To Exercise First Thing...
IN THE MORNING!

Although exercise is profoundly beneficial no matter what time of day you choose to do it, morning exercise rocks! Here are eight great reasons to be an exercise early bird.

1 It begins the day on a positive, "healthy" note that can help set the tone for the rest of the day.

2 It provides an opportunity to tackle and fully complete an activity critical for your health that allows you to begin the day with an immediate sense of accomplishment and empowerment.

3 It increases the chances that you will choose a healthier breakfast. After all, who wants to sabotage a morning workout by following it up with a donut or pastry?

4 It provides an immediate boost in mood and cheerfulness that studies show can last up to 12 hours. (Stand outside the doorway of a gym and watch all the smiling faces upon exit.)

5 It primes the brain for learning and enhances focus in the first one to two hours post-exercise. (Always plan your most cognitively challenging daily activities in the period just after exercise.)

6 It enhances your sleep. Studies show that regular morning exercise improves sleep patterns. In contrast, late afternoon and evening exercise may interfere with sleep onset.

7 Because there are significantly less "competing" events or activities in the earliest parts of the day, morning exercise is easier to build in as a consistent, daily habit. Studies show that early morning exercisers have the best long-term success in maintaining a fitness regimen.

8 It provides a transient increase (up to five hours) in metabolic rate that can help you burn off some of your breakfast and lunch calories. If you do it before your breakfast, you will further maximize fat burning.

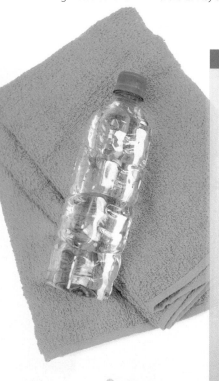

Dr. Ann's...

PLAN OF ACTION

Exercise is a diet pill and an all-round miracle pill that I cannot prescribe with more reverence and enthusiasm—so just do it! To help you get the right exercise for you, here are a few suggestions.

➤ Choose a form of exercise that you like and that fits your lifestyle.

➤ Some good options for most people include: brisk walking, swimming, cycling, or taking advantage of fitness classes or fitness machines in a nearby gym or YMCA.

➤ If you need to, don't be afraid to start with something much less intense like slow walking even a block or two, or down your driveway and back. Even marathon runners begin somewhere and every little bit helps!

➤ If exercise is new for you, remember that it can take up to six months for it to become a habit. Be patient, yet dogged in your daily pursuits. Eventually regular exercise will become an automatic behavior just like brushing your teeth, and that is when you know you are home free!

➤ If the idea of regular exercise just doesn't sit right with you, an alternative is to engage often in lifestyle movement over the day. Examples include sweeping your floors, going up and down steps, raking leaves, shopping on foot, etc.

➤ Always consult with your healthcare provider for an appropriate physical evaluation prior to embarking on any exercise regimen.

“*Perhaps even more exciting, especially for those who prefer moderate activity like brisk walking, even lighter forms of exercise seem to have a beneficial effect on appetite control at the level of the brain.*”

RESEARCH CORNER

Examining Exercise

Whether you prefer a jog in the park or hitting the weight room at the gym, they both seem to help curb over-eating. Researchers at Loughborough University in the United Kingdom had 11 healthy young males engage in three separate experiments to assess the impact of exercise on feelings of hunger and blood levels of appetite-related hormones.

During one session, the study subjects ran on a treadmill for an hour and then rested for seven hours. In another session, they lifted weights for 90 minutes and rested for the next 6 ½ hours. And for the third session, they did no exercise at all. During each of the sessions, the study subjects recorded their feelings of hunger throughout and were provided two separate meals.

In addition, the researchers also measured blood levels of two major appetite hormones, PYY (which decreases appetite) and ghrelin (which increases appetite). During the aerobics session, levels of PYY increased and levels of ghrelin decreased. During the weight-lifting session, levels of ghrelin dropped but levels of PYY remained the same.

The changes in the levels of appetite hormones correlated directly with the study subjects' personal ratings of their own hunger levels. Appetite was suppressed in both the aerobic and weight-lifting sessions over the no-exercise session, but the greatest impact on hunger came from the aerobic exercise session.

Exercise For Appetite Control

Exercise is helpful for weight control on many different fronts and helping you eat less should be added to the list. New research conducted in a group of 18 normal weight and 17 overweight women found that 45 minutes of moderate to vigorous exercise blunted the brain's appetite-stimulating responses to pictures of foods. It is well documented that seeing food images can stimulate the brain's appetite center, and the researchers were curious to see if a bout of exercise could alter the typical response. Both groups of women viewed pictures of appetizing foods after exercise and after a period of quiet rest. In both the normal and overweight women, the brain's responses to food images were reduced after the bout of exercise relative to the period of rest. The investigators also noted that despite the fact that the subjects burned more calories on the day they exercised, they did not compensate by eating additional calories.

Eight Reasons To Exercise If You Want To Lose Weight

❶ Exercise burns belly fat.

❷ Exercise enhances insulin sensitivity (insulin action), which boosts fat burning and reduces fat storage.

❸ Exercise builds lean body mass (muscle). The more muscle mass you have, the more calories you burn all the time.

❹ Exercise reduces stress and anxiety. Stress and anxiety can be powerful triggers for "emotional eating" and binging.

❺ Exercise improves sleep quality and duration. Poor sleep increases appetite and cravings for junk foods. Good sleep enhances self-control and improves energy levels, which means you can eat less and move more!

❻ Exercise directly boosts metabolism. Moderate to vigorous exercise provides a transient (two to five hours) increase in calorie burning potential.

❼ Exercise improves the activity of brain cells involved in appetite regulation.

❽ Exercise improves the release of appetite suppressive hormones in the gastrointestinal tract and the brain's sensitivity to them.

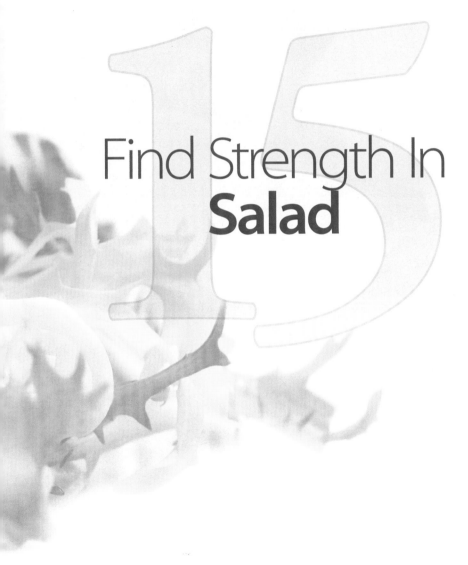

Find Strength In
Salad

Find Strength In
Salad

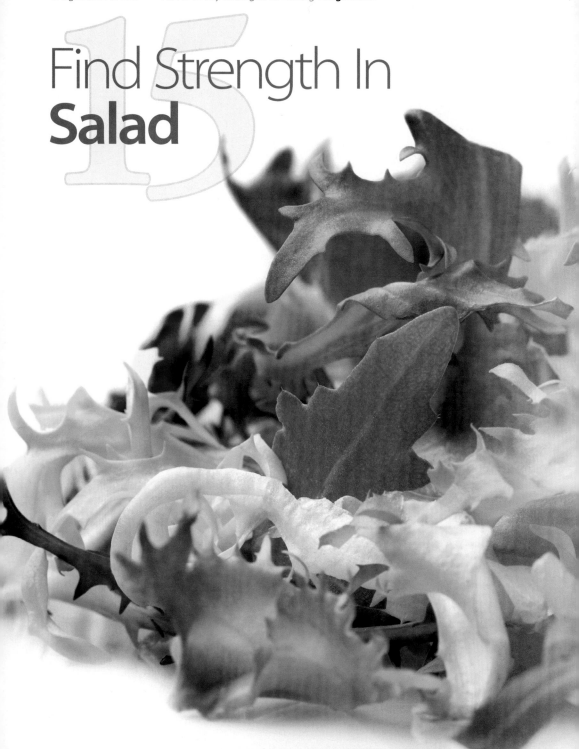

EATING AN ABUNDANCE OF FRUITS AND VEGGIES IS ONE OF THE SUREST WAYS TO BECOME A BIOLOGIC FORTRESS, AND SALADS OFFER AN UNPRECEDENTED OPPORTUNITY TO DAZZLE YOUR TASTE BUDS WITH THIS EXCEPTIONAL FOOD GROUP. Along with sensory pleasure and a total health makeover, salads are also a smart way to help you eat less. Although anytime can be salad time for weight control, research has shown that including a tossed salad as a pre-meal appetizer is an especially helpful way to dial down appetite. In fact, if you dress your salad with a little olive oil-based vinaigrette, this simple mealtime tactic can rein in your appetite in five nifty ways.

First, leafy greens and raw fruits and veggies are rich in fiber. This means their "bulkiness" rapidly fills the stomach and can drive down your hunger hormone, ghrelin, reducing the amount you'll eat for the rest of the meal.

Second, the fat from the olive oil slows stomach emptying, which keeps you feeling fuller longer. Plus, the oleic acid in the olive oil triggers a rapid and more robust release of the "feel-full" hormones from the GI tract.

The vinegar in the dressing plays a role, too. Its acetic acid can hinder digestion by slowing stomach emptying and has even been shown to kick up metabolism a bit. Finally, fiber-rich raw vegetables and fruits require lots of chewing and prolong the eating process. This kicks up orosensory (mouth to brain) satiety and allows more time for your appetite-quieting hormones to do their thing.

Dr. Ann's...
PLAN OF ACTION

To make the most of the appetite-busting benefits of salad, just follow these easy steps:

➤ Enjoy a salad as a pre-meal appetizer.

➤ For best results, strive for 2–3 cups of salad total.

➤ A base of dark green lettuce, like spinach or romaine topped with a variety of brightly colored veggies like carrots, tomatoes, broccoli, bell peppers, and red onions are delicious choices, but go for whatever you like. Fresh fruit can add a delightful sweet touch so do not forget this option.

➤ Dress the salad yourself with a prudent portion (1 to 1 ½ tablespoons) of any olive oil-based vinaigrette. A 3:1 mixture of extra virgin olive oil and balsamic vinegar is an easy option.

➤ Forego the cheese, croutons, bacon bits, and creamy dressings. They will drown out the salad's waist-whittling power.

➤ If prefer your veggies in soup vs. a salad, please note that research also supports that a pre-meal appetizer of a broth-based vegetable soup is also an effective way to help you eat less. So soup it up, as you like.

Research
CORNER

A Study Of Salads

Need more proof that "eating like a rabbit" can lead to weight loss? Consider this. Researchers from Penn State served 42 women an entrée dish of pasta after a pre-meal appetizer of different types of salad or no salad at all. Women who were served 3 cups of a low-calorie salad ate 12% fewer calories overall than those who were not served a salad. Eating 1½ cups of a low-calorie salad reduced the calories the study subjects consumed by 7%. And those provided a high-calorie salad with added cheese and lots of high-fat dressing ate 17% more calories.

The researchers concluded that beginning a meal with a large, low-calorie salad dressed with a prudent portion of dressing (up to about 150 calories) is an effective strategy for curtailing mealtime caloric intake.

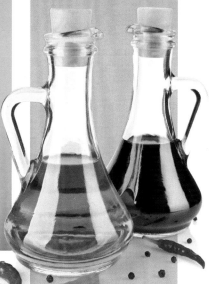

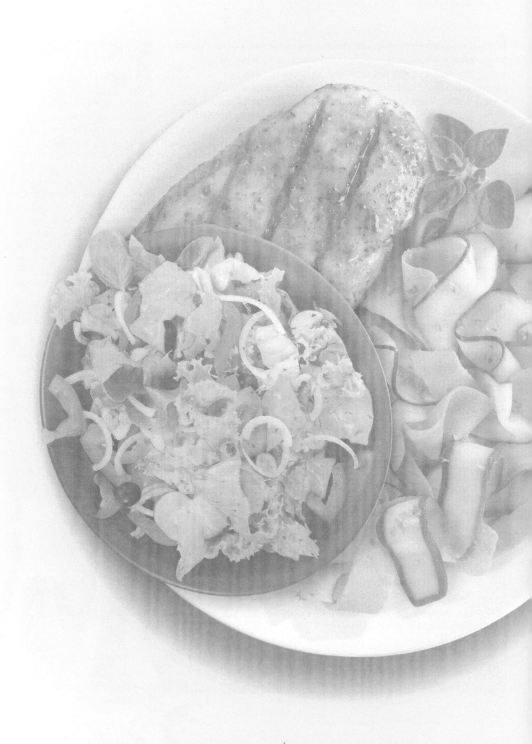

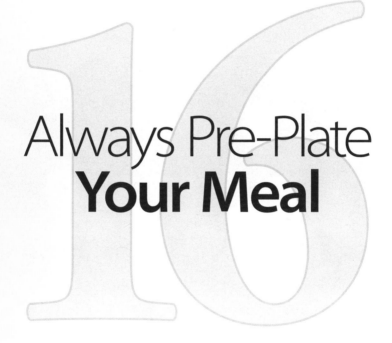

Always Pre-Plate
Your Meal

Always Pre-Plate
Your Meal

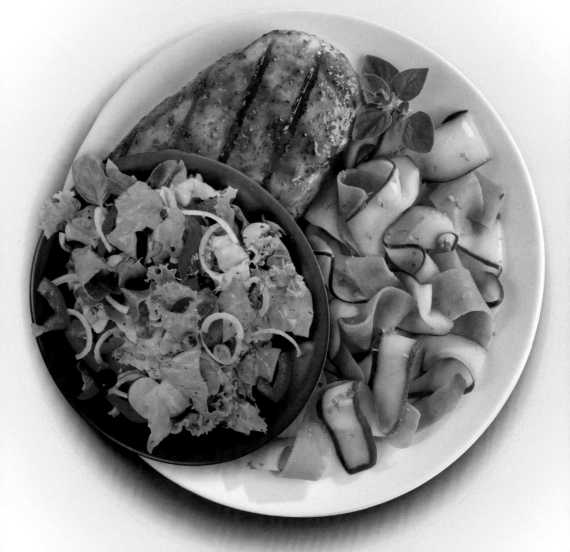

WHETHER IT'S A MEAL, A SNACK, OR A DESSERT—BE VIGILANT ABOUT PRE-PLATING ANY FOOD BEFORE IT CROSSES YOUR LIPS. Studies show that if we can readily view all of our food before and during our indulgences, we tend to eat less. Dr. Brian Wansink, the country's pre-eminent expert on how the external environment influences eating behavior, finds that people eat about 14% less if they pre-plate all the food they intend to eat, rather than serving smaller portions and returning for additional helpings or even worse, consuming the food directly out of its container.

Additionally, seeing food disappear from the plate during consumption serves as a powerful visual cue that eating is progressing and readies you for terminating the meal on a subconscious level. On the other hand, eating directly out of a box, package, or container is especially high-risk for over-eating. Dr. Wansink's studies have confirmed that the less visual perspective we have of the physical quantity of food we are eating—the more we eat regardless of how full we feel.

And of course, being able to preview the entirety of your food on a plate is also essential for practicing portion control. In a country where big dishes bursting with food have unfortunately become the norm, this is paramount for achieving and maintaining a healthy body weight.

Dr. Ann's...
PLAN OF ACTION

The strategy for pre-plating your food really is as easy as it sounds: Don't let anything cross your lips until it has been portioned out on a plate. Here are some additional tips.

➤ Pre-plate not only your meals, but also any snacks and desserts you intend to eat.

➤ Use simple visual cues to achieve the proper portions or serving sizes of different foods. For example, a serving of meat should be about the size of a deck of cards, a serving of nuts the size of a golf ball, a serving of cheese the size of six dice, a serving of oil, salad dressing, or mayo the size of a poker chip, and a serving of dark chocolate the size of a package of dental floss.

➤ Make a concerted effort to specifically look at the food on your plate before you eat it.

➤ Be conscious and visually in-tune with the food leaving your plate and entering your mouth.

Research
CORNER

The Right Dish Matters

To examine the impact of pre-plating, Cornell University's Brian Wansink, PhD, served a group of study subjects a bowl of soup and instructed them to eat until they felt full. One group was served the soup out of a normal bowl, while a second group was served what appeared to them as a normal bowl, but in reality was secretly constructed to remain "bottomless" no matter how much the study subjects ate.

Those with normal bowls ate about 155 calories (about 9 ounces of soup). Those eating from the bottomless bowl ate on average almost twice as much soup—268 calories (15 ounces). Some consumed more than a quart! Even though the bottomless group ate 73% more soup, they reported the same degree of fullness as the regular bowl group.

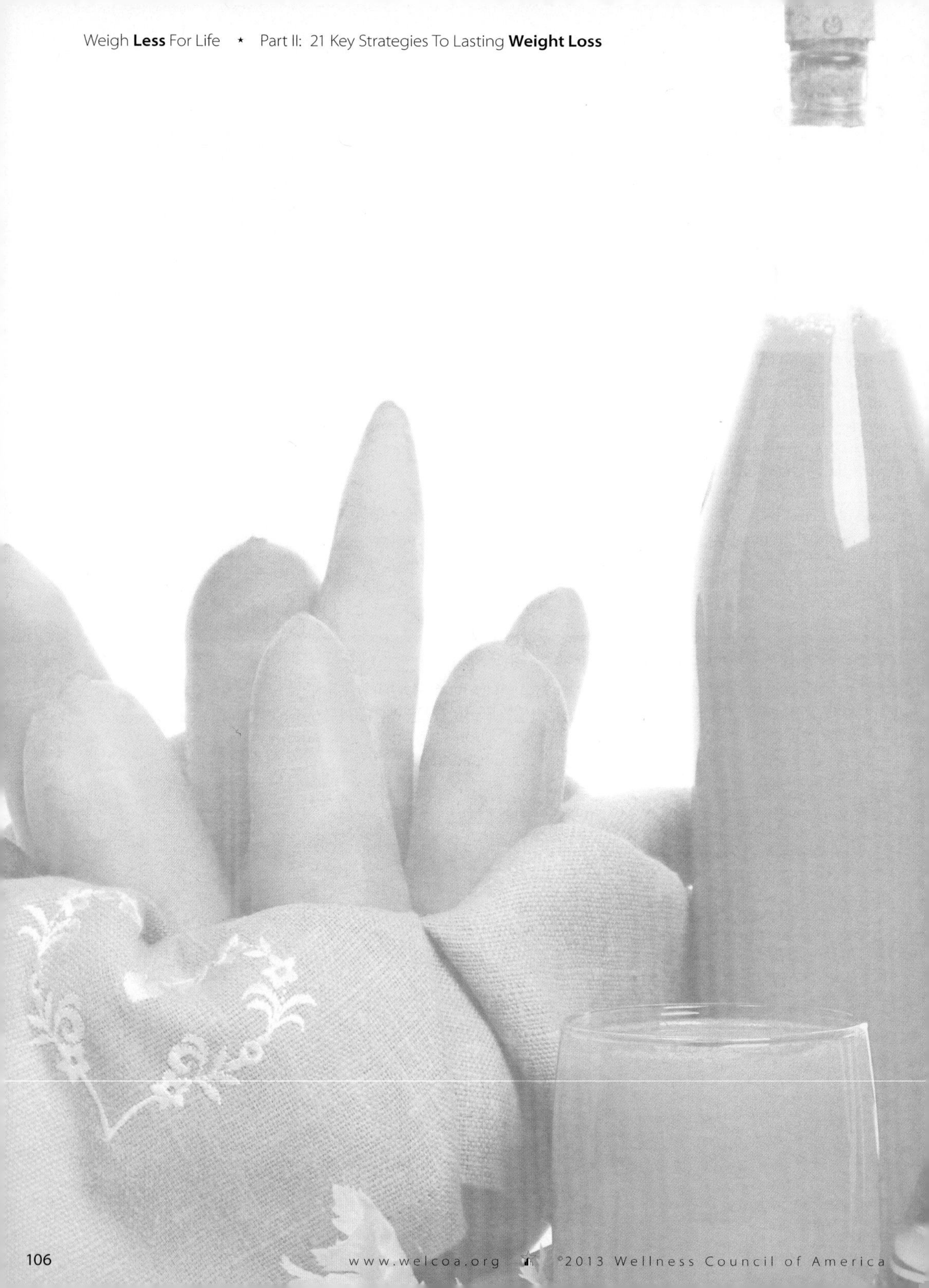

Drink Your
Vegetables

Drink Your
Vegetables

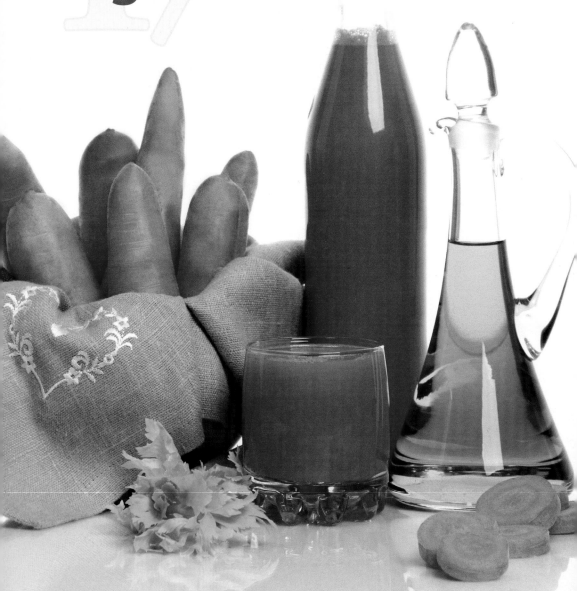

As we learned in a previous chapter, avoiding liquid calories is a fantastic rule to abide by if you want to feel good when you step on the scale. Drinking vegetable juice, however, appears to be a healthy exception.

Vegetables are so steeped in nutrients and so low in calories and sugars that even their juice provides meaningful benefits. Vegetable juices are brimming with vitamins A and C, along with numerous additional heart-healthy plant antioxidants. They also provide a nice dose of potassium—a vital nutrient that most Americans are in dire need of. Thankfully, they provide another key benefit that is in high demand—less hunger. Studies indicate that drinking this wholesome, low-calorie beverage, especially just prior to a meal, helps to reduce your appetite. While scientists aren't exactly sure why, some have speculated that vegetable juices' fiber may take the edge off your hunger. The concentrated supply of nutrients found in vegetable juice might also play a role. Some scientists speculate, me included, that we are driven to eat until we have our "essential" nutrient needs satisfied.

Dr. Ann's...
PLAN OF ACTION

Incorporate vegetable juice into your diet. Even if you don't like vegetable juice, it's worth giving it a try for the benefits it can bring. Here's my best advice for drinking your veggies!

➤ For optimal appetite control, drink 6-8 ounces of vegetable juice just prior to a meal.

➤ Choose a variety you like including tomato juice or the classic V-8, but FORGET the vegetable juice blends that come along with fruit juice like V-8 fusion. They are sugary beverages in disguise!

➤ For the healthiest returns, always opt for the reduced-sodium selections. Many standard vegetable juices are scary-high in sodium.

➤ Of course if you want to juice your own—go for it. I have a juicer for this purpose.

➤ If you're not a fan of vegetable juice, start by trying a little at a time. You'll be pleasantly surprised by how quickly you get used to the taste, and even enjoy it.

➤ And remember that 4 ounces of vegetable juice counts as a full serving of veggies towards your goal of four or more veggie servings a day.

Research CORNER

Vegetable Juice Put To The Test

Researchers at Baylor College of Medicine had 81 study participants who were all following the American Heart Association's DASH diet (Dietary Approaches to Stop Hypertension) drink zero, one, or two 8-ounce cups of low-sodium vegetable juice daily for 12 weeks.

Those who drank the vegetable juice lost an average of four pounds over the course of the 12-week study, while those who didn't lost just one pound. The vegetable juice drinkers also had greater success in meeting their daily requirements of three to five servings of vegetables.

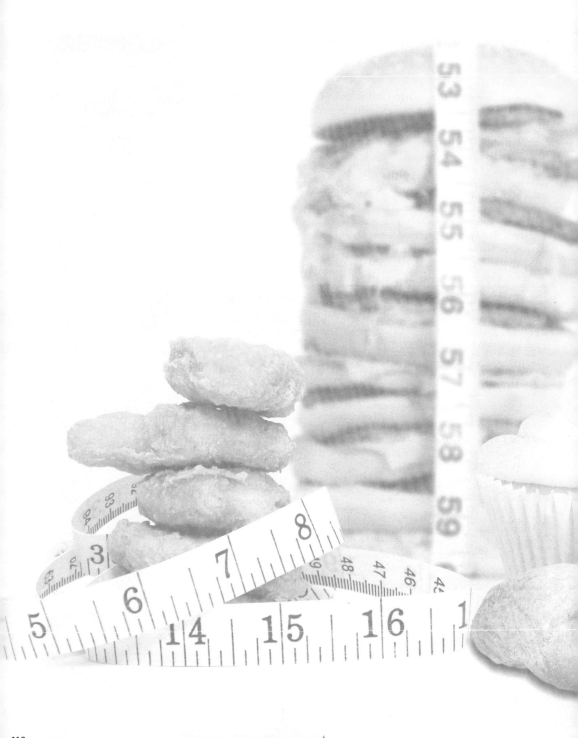

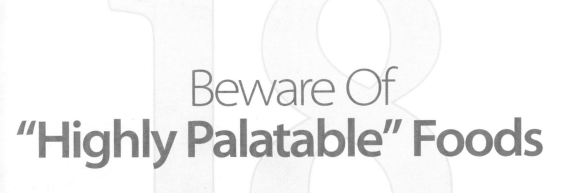

Beware Of
"Highly Palatable" Foods

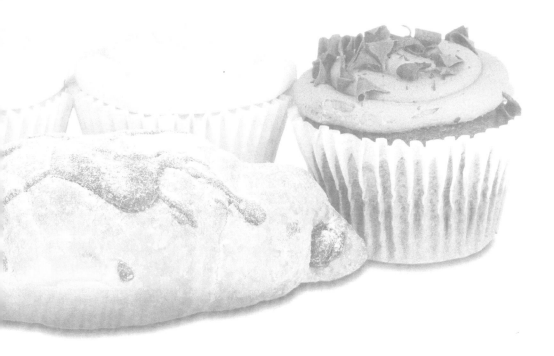

Beware Of
"Highly Palatable" Foods

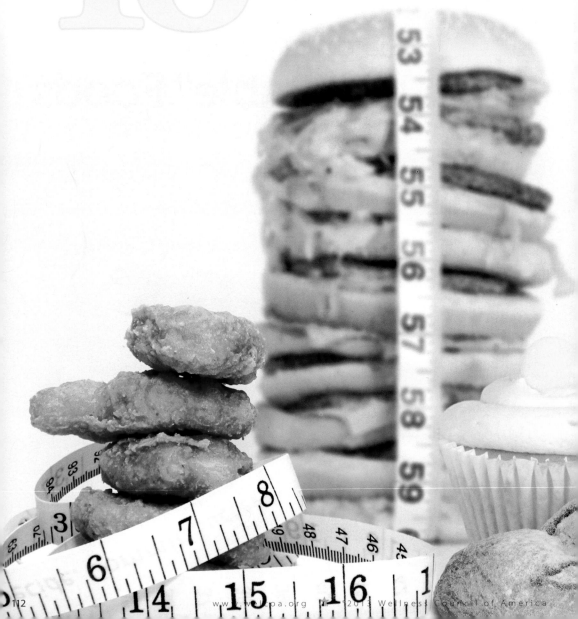

A S HUMANS, OUR TASTE BUDS HAVE A HIGHLY DEVELOPED AND POWERFUL AFFINITY FOR SUGAR, SALT, AND FAT. Combine any two, or better yet all three and our mouths and our brains experience true bliss. This palatal reality developed over the ages because it provided our hunter-gatherer ancestors a valuable survival edge. Sweet and fatty foods were almost always safe to eat, and they provided the most efficient means of bringing in life-sustaining calories and nutrients that were often in short supply.

This was all fine and dandy during the lean and famine-frequent times of our Paleolithic ancestors. Fast-forward to today's world, and the results of these hard-wired palate preferences are disastrous. Let's face it—the American food culture has become a perpetual carnival of sensory delights. Ultra-palatable high-fat, high-sugar foods are literally everywhere, and when we eat them, we want more and more and more.

One of the most provocative advancements in the science of appetite control over the past decade is how a food's flavor and texture profile directly impact the brain. Mounting science is showing that highly flavorful, super-palatable foods (the ones high in sugar, fat, and or salt) can directly stimulate the reward center in the brain. Research in both humans and lab animals shows that once the reward centers are activated by yummy-tasting foods, we will go to great lengths in our attempts to secure another food high. Ultimately, these activating high-fat, high sugar-foods can rewire the brain's appetite control circuitry such that we simply cannot resist them or feel full from them as we should.

Thus the sugar and fat in ultra-palatable foods are "reinforcing" and can lock us into a vicious, self-perpetuating cycle of gluttony that proceeds as follows: eating leads to pleasure leads to desire leads to eating—and so on. This syndrome has been appropriately dubbed "conditioned hypereating." Do not underestimate the powerful lure and addictive potential of sugary and fatty foods!

Fast Food & Depression

Past studies have strongly linked fast food to weight gain, obesity, and type 2 diabetes, and based on a new evaluation it seems we should also add depression to this list. In a long-term study that involved over 8,500 study subjects, those who consumed the most fast food (hamburgers, hot dogs, and pizza) were 51% more likely to develop depression vs. those who rarely or never ate fast food. And there was a direct dose response relationship—the more fast food, the higher the risk, which adds to the likelihood that this could be a direct cause and effect relationship.

As further motivation to keep fast food out of your life and your loved ones' lives—bear in mind that this exceedingly high risk fare houses virtually every single feature scientists have identified that in one way or another leads to overeating. I NEVER eat traditional fast food!

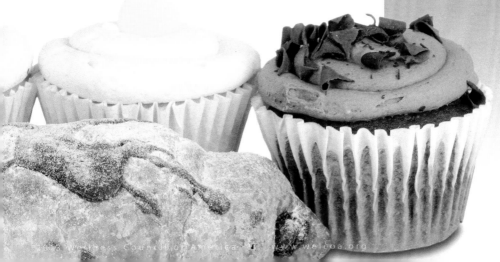

> ❝Do not leave your home hungry. Our external environments are filled with alluring visuals of high risk, bad-for-you foods. Think billboards, fast food signage, etc.❞

Dr. Ann's...
PLAN OF ACTION

It would be easy to tell you to simply avoid these high-fat, high-sugar offenders, but of course, there's a little more to it than that. Here's what I suggest:

➤ Make a concerted effort to reduce your access to and indulgences in foods with a high potential for addiction. Even seeing them can trigger intense cravings at the level of the brain, especially if you are hungry.

➤ The worst offenders are those highest in sugar and fat. The complete list is too lengthy for this book, but some of the worst include: ice cream, milkshakes, pastries, cakes, cookies, donuts, cupcakes, and other sweets/desserts. Bacon cheeseburgers, cheese or regular fries, loaded nachos and potato skins, creamy pasta dishes, and classic fast-food fare are infamous too.

➤ Limit your physical access to these foods by keeping them out of your home and away from your work area. At a minimum, keep them out of sight.

➤ If they somehow make their way into your personal environment and you have any say, be sure they come in small packages. You will eat less chips, cookies, etc. from a small package versus a larger one.

➤ Practice visualizing tantalizing foods with a stream of negative, even repulsive images. Overtime this can help you say no to them more readily.

➤ Use personally empowered language like "I don't" versus "I can't" or "no" when refusing highly-palatable foods. This simple verbal maneuver can be highly effective.

➤ Perhaps the easiest way to safeguard your waistline from these provocative foods is to stick to Mother Nature's fare. The subtle and simpler flavor profiles in whole, natural foods will satisfy you without zapping your pleasure centers and overriding your self-control.

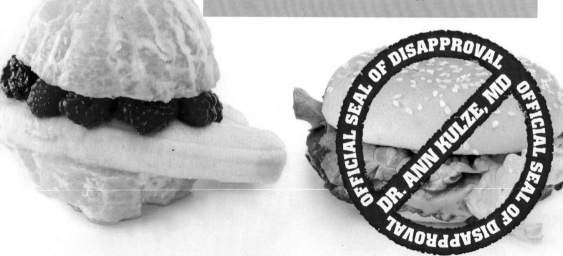

OFFICIAL SEAL OF DISAPPROVAL
DR. ANN KULZE, MD
OFFICIAL SEAL OF DISAPPROVAL

RESEARCH CORNER

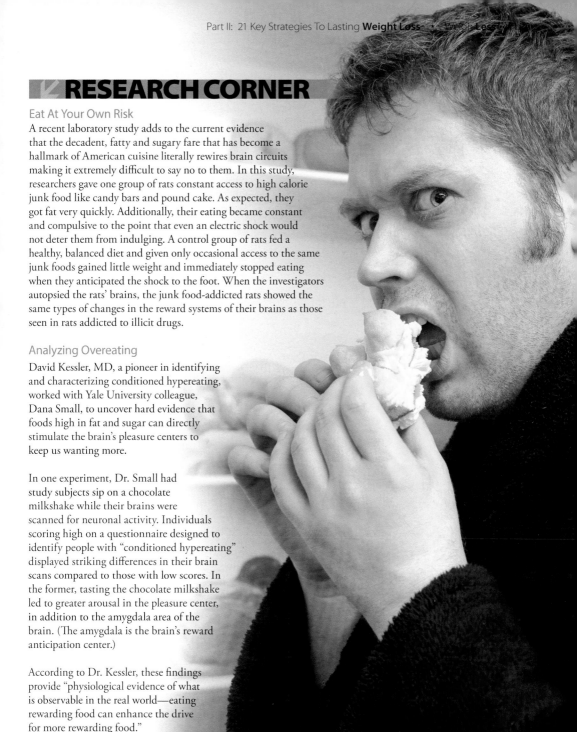

Eat At Your Own Risk

A recent laboratory study adds to the current evidence that the decadent, fatty and sugary fare that has become a hallmark of American cuisine literally rewires brain circuits making it extremely difficult to say no to them. In this study, researchers gave one group of rats constant access to high calorie junk food like candy bars and pound cake. As expected, they got fat very quickly. Additionally, their eating became constant and compulsive to the point that even an electric shock would not deter them from indulging. A control group of rats fed a healthy, balanced diet and given only occasional access to the same junk foods gained little weight and immediately stopped eating when they anticipated the shock to the foot. When the investigators autopsied the rats' brains, the junk food-addicted rats showed the same types of changes in the reward systems of their brains as those seen in rats addicted to illicit drugs.

Analyzing Overeating

David Kessler, MD, a pioneer in identifying and characterizing conditioned hypereating, worked with Yale University colleague, Dana Small, to uncover hard evidence that foods high in fat and sugar can directly stimulate the brain's pleasure centers to keep us wanting more.

In one experiment, Dr. Small had study subjects sip on a chocolate milkshake while their brains were scanned for neuronal activity. Individuals scoring high on a questionnaire designed to identify people with "conditioned hypereating" displayed striking differences in their brain scans compared to those with low scores. In the former, tasting the chocolate milkshake led to greater arousal in the pleasure center, in addition to the amygdala area of the brain. (The amygdala is the brain's reward anticipation center.)

According to Dr. Kessler, these findings provide "physiological evidence of what is observable in the real world—eating rewarding food can enhance the drive for more rewarding food."

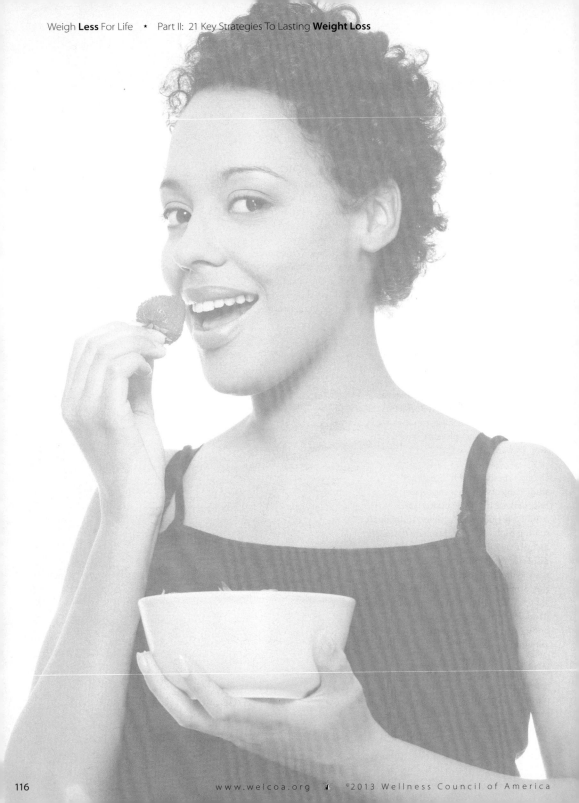

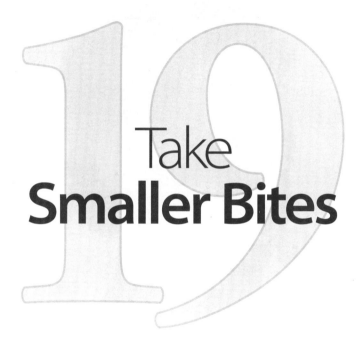

Take
Smaller Bites

Take
Smaller Bites

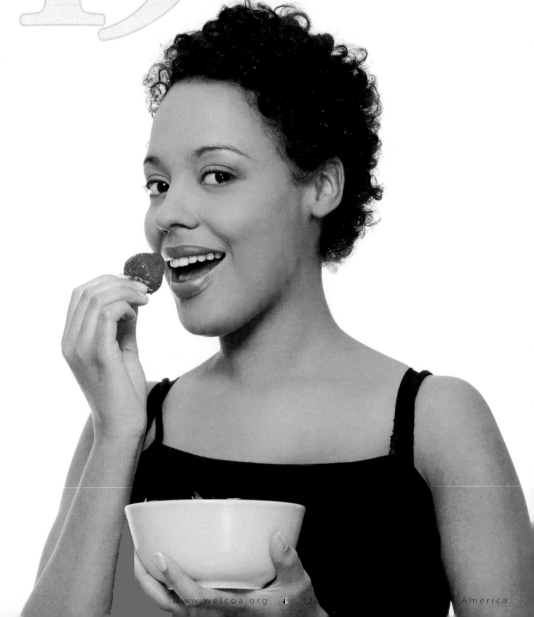

www.welcoa.org

Taking smaller bites is perhaps the simplest strategy of all to help you eat less. The reason this tip works is elementary: The more oral exposure you have to the food in a meal or a snack, the better your appetite suppression will be. As mentioned in previous chapters, the mouth is loaded with sensory receptors that are hardwired directly into the brain's appetite control center. The more those receptors can directly engage with the specific tastes and textures in a food, the stronger and more abundant the "fullness" signals will be that your mouth relays to your brain.

In addition to providing a greater feeling of fullness through sensory signals, taking smaller bites also prolongs the time it will take you to finish eating. Remember, it takes a full 20 minutes for appetite-suppressive hormones to be released after food enters your stomach. By taking your time and eating slowly, you give those hormones the time they need to reach and quiet the brain's hunger sensor, which will help you stop eating when you're actually full!

Dr. Ann's...
PLAN OF ACTION

If you're not accustomed to taking small bites, it can take a little bit of time to get the hang of it. These tips will help.

➤ Make a conscious, concerted effort to take smaller bites of food.

➤ Be mindful of each and every small bite you take to savor and enjoy the flavors, and textures in each chew.

➤ Downsize to smaller eating utensils. The smaller your fork or spoon - the more apt you are to reduce your bite size.

➤ Eat more high fiber, unprocessed foods like whole fruits and vegetables. Their physical structure naturally encourages smaller bites and slower chewing.

➤ Use food aroma enhancers like onions, garlic, cinnamon, rosemary, curry and other herbs and spices liberally in your meals and dishes. The more powerful a food's aroma, the smaller bites we tend to take.

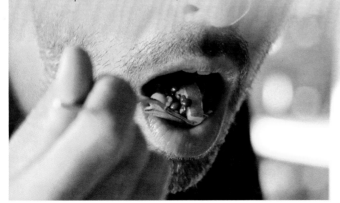

Research
CORNER

Science You Can Sink Your Teeth Into

Even a step as simple as taking smaller bites of food has science on its side. In the Netherlands, researchers fed 22 healthy subjects a portion of chocolate custard during two separate experiments. In the first experiment, the bite sizes of the participants were limited to 5 grams. Then, for the second experiment, the subjects were allowed to take bites as large as 15 grams.

During both experiments, the study subjects were told to eat as much custard as they desired. Not surprisingly, the subjects ate on average 28% less custard when they consumed it in smaller bites.

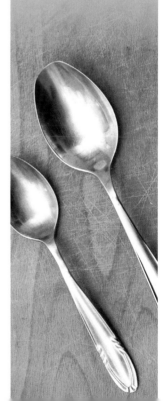

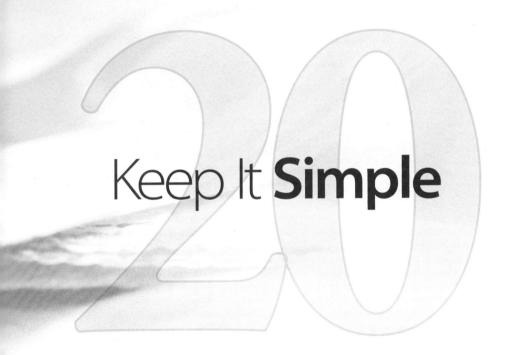

Keep It **Simple**

Keep It
Simple

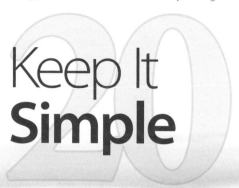

Variety may be the spice of life, but with your foods, variety can bring on the fat.

It's a scientific fact: The greater the variety or selection of food choices we have, the more we tend to order or serve ourselves, and ultimately the more we eat. The basis for this behavioral trait likely stems from our dependence on a broad range of essential nutrients distributed amongst a vast array of different foods. Eating a variety of foods would have provided our ancestors a better chance of survival. On top of this instinctive trait, in the face of a variety of foods, we perceive lesser quantities of each of them than are actually present. This visual trick leads us to help ourselves to larger servings without realizing it. Compounding things further—variety also diminishes our sense of food satisfaction, which provides us with even further inducement to eat more. Given this trifecta of vulnerability in concert with our modern food landscapes that are now so filled with options and variety that our heads spin—the risk for over-eating abounds.

Take home message: The perils of dining variety in concert with our genes underscore how important it is to limit exposures to an abundance of food or meal choices if we want to control our weight!

KEEP IT STEADY-EDDIE

Keeping your appetite under wraps can be as simple as maintaining your blood glucose level. Here is my best advice for preventing those hunger-driving drops in your blood glucose.

❶ Minimize foods known to precipitously drop your blood sugar—namely, the refined, high glycemic "Great White Hazards"—white flour products, white potatoes, white rice and sugar/sweets. Sugary beverages, sweets, and white potatoes are the worst offenders! These three categories of carbs can actually drive blood glucose levels down below what is physiologically normal. Eating these "bad carbs" can perpetuate the vicious cycle of low glucose > cravings > more bad carbs > low glucose > more cravings, etc.

❷ Eat three meals daily with a mid-afternoon snack. Eating the right foods is what sustains a normal blood glucose level. It's especially important to always eat breakfast, as skipping breakfast has been associated with increased food cravings.

❸ Be sure to have some healthy protein at each meal. Protein provides a stable and more prolonged blood glucose level. If you are hungry (a dead ringer indicator of low blood glucose) within 2 ½ hours of a meal, you likely did not eat enough protein. A reasonable amount to aim for is 20 to 25 grams per meal.

❹ Regularly include the super nutritious and healthy "slower carbs" in your meals—physically intact whole grains, beans, fruits and veggies (not white potatoes). Because of their lack of processing and high fiber content they provide a more stable blood glucose response.

❺ Avoid artificially sweetened beverages, especially all by themselves. Artificial sweeteners are exquisitely sweet substances that may trigger the release of insulin, which lowers blood sugar!

> Keep convenient Ziploc bags filled with finger-friendly cut up veggies in a high-profile spot in your fridge. Put a large bowl brimming with brightly colored fruits right on your kitchen counter or work desk.

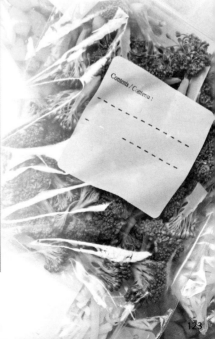

Dr. Ann's...
PLAN OF ACTION

Luckily, "keeping it simple" doesn't mean that you're locked into a life of boring, limited food choices. Here's what I suggest to enjoy food responsibly.

➤ **Limit dining out.** Restaurants, especially fast food joints, are home to a vast and ever-growing menu of different food options. My best advice is to never set foot in any traditional fast food restaurants.

➤ **Avoid buffet lines and all-you-can-eat cafeterias.** Seeing the actual foods in such a dazzling array of options poses the greatest risk for over-indulgence.

➤ **Strive to prepare and eat most of your foods from home.** Brown bag it for lunch and or breakfast as needed.

➤ **Turn the "eat more in the face of variety" to your advantage by keeping a variety of healthy fruits and veggies as visible and as available as possible at all times.** Keep convenient Ziploc bags filled with finger-friendly cut up veggies in a high-profile spot in your fridge. Put a large bowl brimming with brightly colored fruits right on your kitchen counter or work desk.

RESEARCH CORNER

The Science Of Simple
A number of studies on different topics have explored an interesting phenomenon: Seeing a variety of objects in one location leads to the false perception that each object occupies less space. Naturally, investigators were curious if the same perception would occur with food.

To test that theory, researchers instructed 105 study participants to pour a certain amount of M&M's from a clear, 32-ounce container into four separate 6-inch bowls. Participants were first allowed to practice using brown M&M's until they were confident with the amount that they were being asked to pour.

After the practice session, study participants were given a container of M&M's in a single color or an even mixture of three colors and instructed to pour the same amount from the practice session into four bowls. Study subjects poured significantly more candy (up to 30% more) from the container that had the multi-colored M&M's than they did from the container that held the single-colored M&M's. The study confirmed that people serve up bigger portions when provided with more variety.

Dr. Ann's Favorite Tips On...
STRESS RELIEF

Stress is bad to the belly. Here are some tips to help you stay cool and trim.

➤ **Move.** Commit to walking briskly for 30 minutes or more daily (the more the better). Physical activity relieves stress, lifts mood, dissipates anxiety, and improves sleep. The "cross pattern" repetitive movement of walking has been shown to have a unique calming effect on the brain. Even better, do your walking in a beautiful natural setting (the beach, a park, etc). Gazing out in natural settings has been shown to provide immediate stress reduction. This interesting psychological phenomenon has been dubbed "biophilia."

➤ **Get in a good laugh.** Rent your favorite comedy movies or reruns of funny sitcoms. Watch some funny YouTube videos with friends or family. Laughing is fun and lowers levels of stress hormones. If you can't laugh, at least put a smile on your face. Smiling instantly induces relaxation.

➤ **Sip on some hot, freshly brewed tea.** This relaxing and healthy ritual has been shown to help lower stress hormones in the body.

➤ **Listen to music with a slow or meditative tempo.** This can facilitate relaxation.

➤ **Get hot!** Throw some hot spices (chili pepper) or condiments into your foods. Hot foods stimulate the pain receptors in the mouth, which triggers the release of endorphins. Endorphins are the body's "natural" morphine-like chemicals that promote feelings of euphoria and enhanced well-being.

➤ **Get a foot massage or better yet, a whole body massage.** They feel great, help you relax, and improve blood flow.

➤ **Twice a day (or when you feel anxious or stressed), take a two to three minute break from life and calm yourself by deep breathing as follows:**

- Exhale slowly and completely through your mouth.
- Inhale slowly and deeply through your nose to a count of five with your mouth closed.
- Hold your breath to a count of five.
- Exhale slowly through your mouth to a count of seven.
- Repeat for a total of four or more breaths.

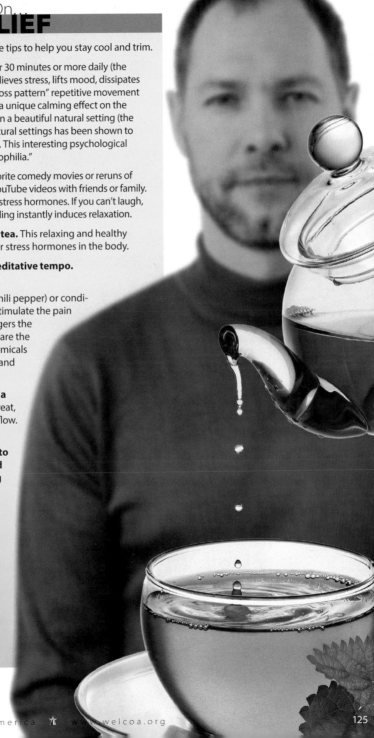

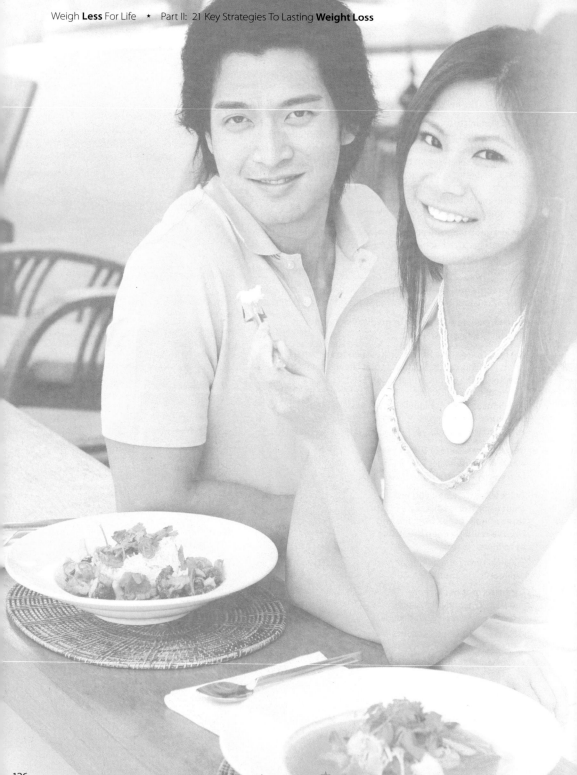

Slow Down And **Enjoy!**

Slow Down And
Enjoy!

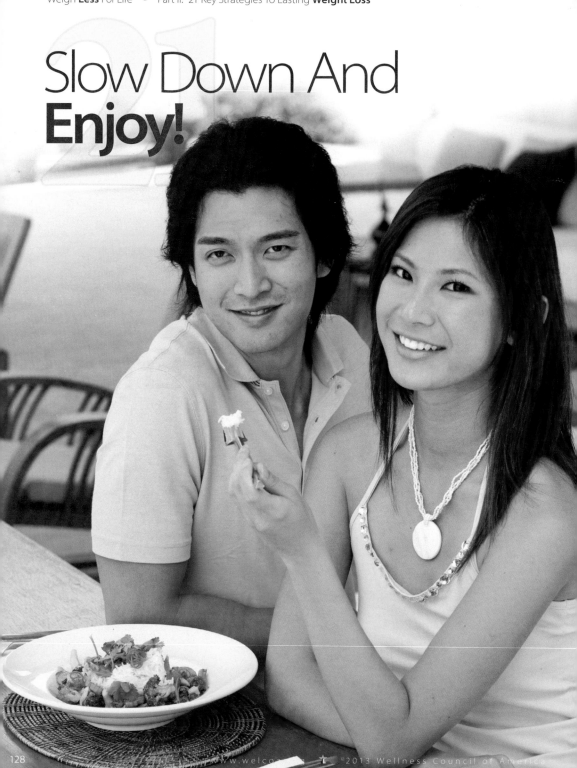

Stand Up To Sitting!

Regardless of how active you are or how much you exercise, prolonged sitting is an independent risk factor for weight gain, metabolic dysfunction, osteoporosis, and some cancers. Here are my tips to stand up to sitting!

► Transition to a stand up desk—I have one and LOVE it!

► Drink enough water during the day that you will need to get up and urinate every two hours.

► Set your watch, phone, or computer to beep at regular intervals to remind you to get up and move. If I know my day will involve mostly sitting (like when I write), I try to stand up every hour and do jumping jacks for one minute.

► Make all your phone calls standing up.

► Keep your office trash can and office fax machine a few feet away from your desk to force you to get up to use them.

► Strive to move during your leisure time—do not sit during times away from your office desk.

► Limit TV viewing, and get up and move during commercial breaks.

► Stand up during office meetings or better yet conduct meetings during a walk.

► Walk around during your lunch break.

► Be grateful for after work household chores that require you to move.

► Be aware that the most important times to avoid prolonged sitting are in the immediate one to two hours after eating.

► Strive for three minutes of activity for every one hour you are sitting. Even light activity is beneficial.

A S IT TURNS OUT, YOUR MOTHER'S CONSTANT REQUESTS TO, "SLOW DOWN" AND "CHEW YOUR FOOD" HAD SOUND SCIENTIFIC REASONING BEHIND THEM. The research is compelling—the faster we eat, the more food we consume.

Studies have shown that wolfing down a meal thwarts the body's innate appetite-control process and leads to greater food intake. When food enters the stomach, a number of hormones are released from the gut that stifle the appetite signals emanating from your brain's hunger center. It takes a full 20 minutes for these satiety (make-me-feel-full) signals to reach and to begin quieting the brain's hunger sensor. Additionally, there is evidence that the faster you eat, the lower the levels of appetite-suppressive hormones your gut releases. Eating at a leisurely pace allows ample time for your body's natural feel-full signals to reach their peak and fully kick in. Deliberate slow eating with focused attention on each bite of food also naturally encourages "mindfulness." Growing science is finding mindfulness-based eating highly effective for weight control.

In today's get-it-done-now, sped-up world, clearly there's one thing that we should take our time with—and that's eating. So the next time you feel the urge to rush through a meal, just stop, take a few deep breaths to relax, and enjoy instead. Your waistline and your peace of mind are both sure to benefit.

Dr. Ann's PLAN OF ACTION

The secret to eating less in this case is simple—slow down and savor! To help you with that, here are a few simple rules to adhere to.

► Spend at least 20 minutes eating each meal. If you can spend more time, it's even better.

► NEVER go back for second helpings until it has been at least 20 minutes from your first bite.

► Take the time to chew and relish each and every bite. As you chew, focus on each bite for its flavors, textures, and aromas. In other words, practice mindfulness when you eat.

► Reserve eating for eating. Strive to eat all of your meals from a table without the presence of distracting influences like the TV or a computer. Mindless eating in front of the TV is notorious for overconsumption!

► Make the effort to join others at mealtime whenever possible and engage in conversation. Chatting between bites can really help slow things down.

► Develop the habit of purposely putting your fork down and removing your hands from it between each bite.

► Remember that speed eating equals overeating!

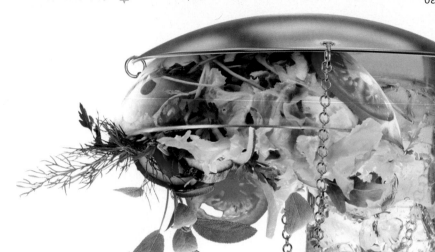

Weigh Less, **Be More**

THANK YOU FOR THE PLEASURE OF ALLOWING ME TO GUIDE YOU DOWN THE HEALTHY AND RELIABLE PATH OF *WEIGH LESS FOR LIFE*. Armed with the 21 strategies in the preceding pages, I know you can rein in your hunger and become the ultimate ruler of what and how much you eat. I also know that you can depend on these very same strategies to transform your health for the better, both for yourself, as well as for the people who love you. In addition, I've included my *Weigh Less, Be More Scorecard* (on the next page) as a tool to help you track your progress.

Always remember that YOU are the only person that can make YOU healthy and that controlling your weight is one of the single most powerful tools you have for guarding your health and maintaining your vitality. As you continue on your rewarding weigh less journey, I would love to hear from you and welcome your feedback at **www.DrAnnWellness.com.**

If you want additional wellness motivation and education, I have a full library of free resources available from my website including: video tips, articles, podcasts, and much more. For the latest and greatest in health and nutrition news, sign up for my bi-weekly Dr. Ann's Wellness Bulletin, and follow me on Twitter: @**DrAnnWellness,** Facebook, and Instagram.

Lastly, I am grateful to my good friends at the Wellness Council of America (WELCOA) for bringing my guidance for better health and weight control to life with this visually captivating and warmly engaging book. On behalf of both of us, we wish you the very best in all of your wellness endeavors and are always cheering you on in spirit!